# WORKING THROUGH THE DARK

ASANTE CLEVELAND WITH JORDAN PINCKNEY

# COPYRIGHT

# ACKNOWLEDGEMENTS

There have been so many people in my life who have played some role (both big and small) to help me get to where I am now. I cannot overlook them and the brightness they brought to my heart.

To my parents, thank you for teaching me the values of working hard and seeing myself as more than just an athlete. Thank you for revealing the value of compassion and kindness. You showed me the importance of holding onto true character.

To all of my coaches, I cannot thank you enough for the lessons you instilled in my mind and craft. I cannot thank you enough for believing in me when I didn't yet  believe in myself. You saw something I hadn't seen, and I thank you all for never giving up on me.

To all my former teammates, I am so grateful to have been able to compete with you and alongside you. I am thankful for our experiences and friendships both on the field and off the field. We went through the hardships of competition. Thank you for those journeys.

To Joseph, thank you so much for encouraging me to share my story, as well as connecting me with Jordan.

To Coach Mangini, thank you for your friendship and

guidance through the years. Thank you for taking the time to be my beta reader. Your football wisdom was just as invaluable as the life wisdom you shared throughout our years together. (Also, a special shout out to Jake. Thanks for being a beta reader.)

To Alex and Kent, thank you for giving valuable feedback in my story and we worked hard through it from cover to cover. Your insight was so helpful and it brought the best effort into making this story be told the best way possible.

To Will Lenzen Junior, thank you for putting together the goal post, because it helped display the vision of the book and articulate the message I wanted to pass on to the reader. Thank you for taking time away from your projects to be a part of mine. (Check out his nonprofit at createecho.org)

To Kris, thank you so much for your efficient work despite having a baby boy, working odd hours to make this vision happen, and putting your passion into this project. I am so grateful that you were willing to showcase your artwork to tell my story.  (You can find his work @kriswantowhy on Instagram)

To Ajao, thank you so much for your patience and your diligence. Thank you for your commitment to this project. Your help to organize and format this book reveals your craftsmanship. You can find his work at https://www.behance.net/ajaoifeolua95d

To Aubree, thank you so much for making sense of my ideas, and then magically turning them into coherent thoughts. It was your patience and attention to detail that brought precision to the book. I am grateful for your time and expertise.

To Bethany, thank you for helping me discover the flow to this story. I full-heartedly appreciate your perseverance as you dealt with the loss of a loved one. You have such a loving heart to put time into our project while also moving across the state of Iowa for your new job. (You can find her work at bjpeat.com)

To Jordan, thank you for your timeless work and effort to help me tell my story. I appreciate your background, perspective, and genuine desire to help me make a difference. I'm grateful that you brought in many people onto this project to make this dream a reality.

# CONTENTS

# POEMS

## 'IF'
### *By Rudyard Kipling*

If you can keep your head when all about you
Are losing theirs and blaming it on you,
If you can trust yourself when all men doubt you,
But make allowance for their doubting too;
If you can wait and not be tired by waiting,
Or being lied about, don't deal in lies,
Or being hated, don't give way to hating,
And yet don't look too good, nor talk too wise:

If you can dream—and not make dreams your master;
If you can think—and not make thoughts your aim;
If you can meet with Triumph and Disaster
And treat those two impostors just the same;
If you can bear to hear the truth you've spoken
Twisted by knaves to make a trap for fools,
Or watch the things you gave your life to, broken,

And stoop and build 'em up with worn-out tools:

If you can make one heap of all your winnings
And risk it on one turn of pitch-and-toss,
And lose, and start again at your beginnings
And never breathe a word about your loss;
If you can force your heart and nerve and sinew
To serve your turn long after they are gone,
And so hold on when there is nothing in you
Except the Will which says to them: 'Hold on!'

If you can talk with crowds and keep your virtue,
Or walk with Kings—nor lose the common touch,
If neither foes nor loving friends can hurt you,
If all men count with you, but none too much;
If you can fill the unforgiving minute
With sixty seconds' worth of distance run,
Yours is the Earth and everything that's in it,
And—which is more—you'll be a Man, my son!

**IX**

# 'INVICTUS'

*By William Earnest Henley*

Out of the night that covers me,
Black as the pit from pole to pole,
I thank whatever gods may be
For my unconquerable soul.

In the fell clutch of circumstance
I have not winced nor cried aloud.
Under the bludgeonings of chance
My head is bloody, but unbowed.

Beyond this place of wrath and tears
Looms but the Horror of the shade,
And yet the menace of the years
Finds and shall find me unafraid.

It matters not how strait the gate,
How charged with punishments the scroll,
I am the master of my fate,
I am the captain of my soul.

X

# WARNING

Note to the reader:
This book contains descriptive events from Asante's life,
some of which may be difficult to read at times.

# 1

# THE DARK

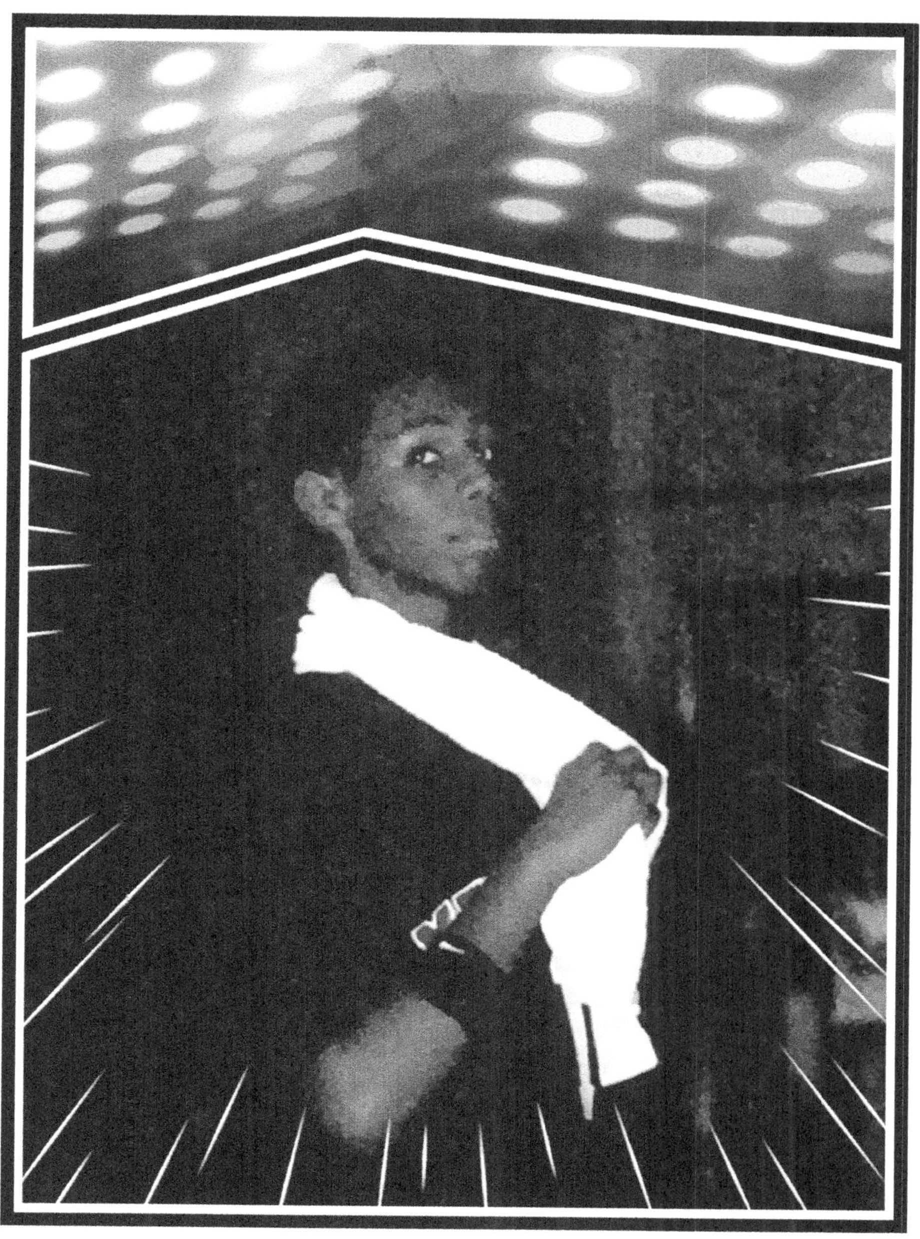

ask myself every day how much abuse shaped me. Whenever I look in the mirror, I wonder who that man would have been if my childhood was normal. It's a complicated thought. What is normal? When I reflect on where I came from and who I am now, I can't help but wonder, would I have made it to the NFL if my childhood had been different? As a kid, if I had known where my future would end up, would the abuse have been easier for me to endure?

When I ponder my past, present, and future, I realize something. I can't answer these questions, because they aren't the right questions. The answers won't solve anything or change anything. They can't teach me anything new about myself. They are just empty questions I have fixated on for too long. So, what is the right question? In order to find out, I need to reflect on how I grew. Like a seed, I started in the dirt; broken open and reaching for the light. William Ernest Henley writes from his poem, "Invictus":

> *Out of the night that covers me,*
> *Black as the pit from pole to pole,*
> *I thank whatever gods may be*
> *For my unconquerable soul.*

Starting at age five, I was forced to endure years

of undeserved punishment at the hands of my abuser. For most of those years, no one had any idea what was happening to me. Some people would be surprised to learn that I don't hate Her. Her actions could have destroyed me, and I could have let them. I would be justified to take out all of my anger on my abuser, and make Her feel as small and nonexistent as I felt, but that would be giving up my super power. I refuse to let go of the strength I earned through surviving her abuse. I choose instead to thank Her for what I can. I will thank Her for revealing to me that I was made of much more than she saw, or said, or showed. She wounded my body, and tried to crush my mind; but I created my spirit.

Do I hold the trauma I experienced against her? That's one of the *right* questions, and the answer to that is 'no.' Because in the darkness, where I felt completely alone, something was growing inside of me. Deep down, beneath all of that anger and hate and confusion, the seed began to sprout into who I am today.

Every human being lives and experiences struggles, situations, and successes differently from each other. Our lives are incomparable. Sure, some things can be similar. That's how we connect relationally and socially, but there are no two stories that are truly the same. That's what makes us unique. That's what makes us individuals. Hundreds of millions of stories are never told. When I hear

someone's life story, I see the lessons threaded within —
like a spider web of knowledge and teachings. But there are
so many strands never told, never revealed, never exposed.
They just stay hidden in the dark.

It can be disheartening to think about. So many
people who never tell their story, who never reflect on
their life. We *all* have something to share about ourselves,
something to offer one another. I have a story. You have a
story. The bus driver has a story. But something keeps us
from sharing.

Why? And why has it taken *me* so long to share
mine? That's another right question. As you read my story,
I hope it encourages you to think about your own life. I
didn't write this book because I thought I was special. No,
I wrote this because I know it can help someone see their
own potential, maybe even you. You *also* have a seed that
is growing. I want you to see it. And I want you to know, I'm
here for you. I got your back. And I know there is greatness
inside of you, even if you don't see it yet.

Hello, my name is Asante Cleveland, and I played in
the NFL. But that's not the story I want to tell. My story
isn't about what happened under the stadium lights, but
about what came out of the dark.

# 2

# THE LESSON

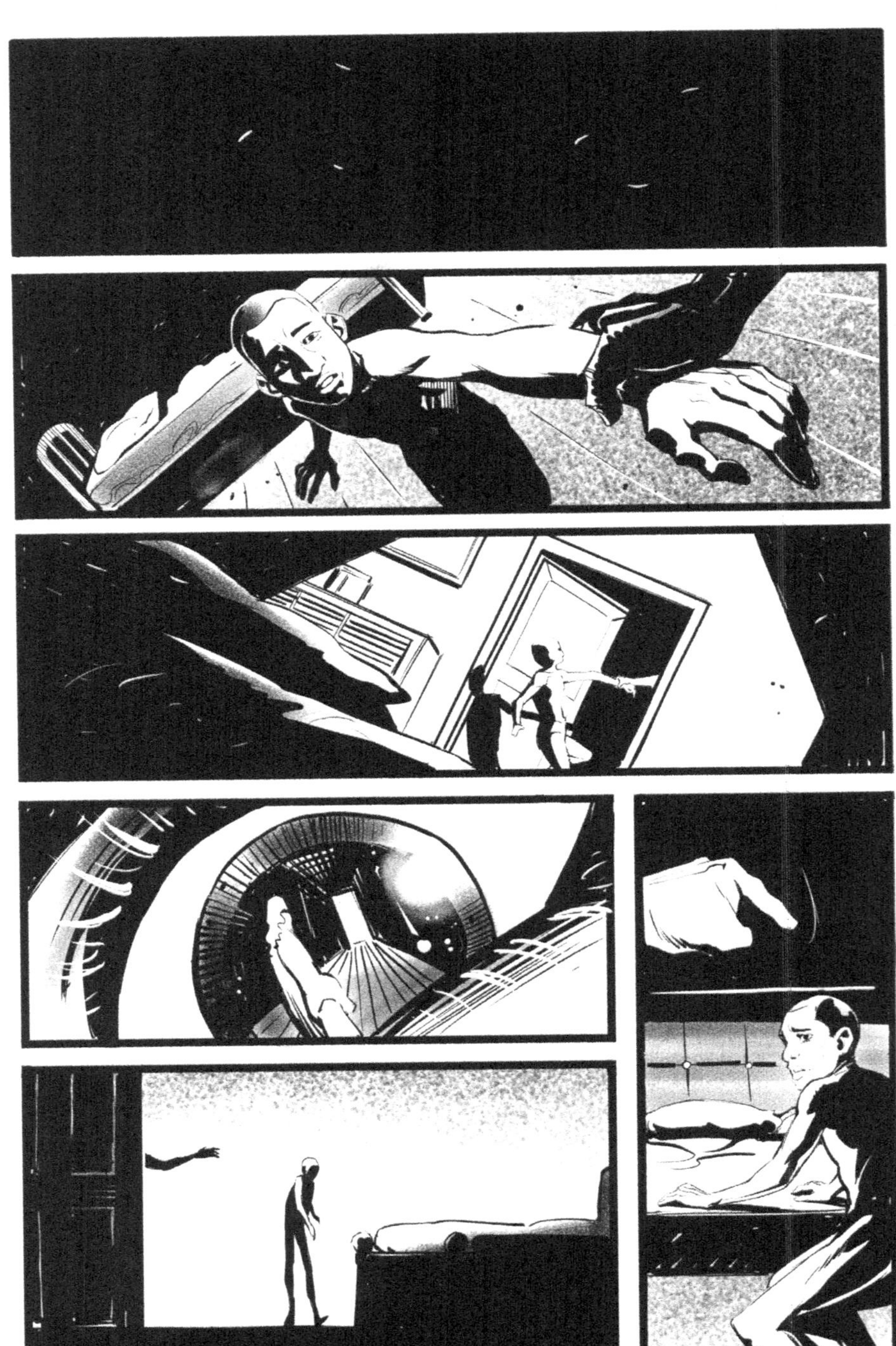

**"**Get up."

The bone-chilling sound of my abuser's voice woke me from a dead sleep. I was instantly bathed in terror and crushing disappointment.

My eleven-year-old self had gone to bed so sure I had done it. I had escaped her wrath this time and had made it to my bed without her noticing my small mistake hours earlier. She had allowed me to sleep, luring me into a false sense of security, but it was clear now that I had been gravely mistaken.

I thought I was getting better at seeing the signs of her rage. I was learning to predict when wrath would rain down on me, and I recognized her routine of unleashing that rage. Going to bed, last night, I had thought I'd successfully avoided setting off the fury inside her. I felt I had won a small victory.

Sleep had come easily to me for the first time in a long while. I had breathed freely and slept deep enough to dream.

But I was dead wrong. The inevitable had only been delayed.

"Get up," She hissed, as she yanked my underwear-clad body from my bed and pulled me down the dark hallway. The peace I had felt had already fled into the shadows, hiding where I could not.

She squeezed me through the doorway of her bedroom and pushed me towards her bed. "Lay down."

Disobedience wasn't an option. I was unable to think as I crawled onto her bed and lay flat on my back. I knew what was coming.

She left the room and a sinister hush fell over me. The entire room was shrouded in silence. The calm before the storm. In the quiet, my mind began to work. I could hear every step, every breath, and every drawer that opened and slammed shut in the other room.

Propping up on my elbows, I thought wildly about escaping, but the only way out was through her bedroom door. Impossible. She was out there, looking for something I prayed she wouldn't find. What she searched for had been loaned to us by a helpful neighbor years ago and never returned. Instead, it had been molded into a weapon of torment to use against me. My ears followed her every step as she shuffled around in the dark.

Shivers of anxiety crawled their way through my nervous system as the chilly air cooled my sweaty skin. There was another unmistakable sound of a drawer opening, then a hesitation before it slammed shut. I knew she had found it, and my heart rocketed into my throat.

The pounding of her returning footsteps echoed the

pounding pulse in my ears. The punisher approached and there was no one to save me. There was no last stand or overtime. This was the inevitable moment that I had experienced so many times. She ruled me, both mentally and emotionally, and she knew it. I was powerless.

Seconds slowed as I heard the dreaded sound of rubbery plastic slapping sickly on her palm. She had found the twelve-inch-long glue stick, and she was bringing it back to the bedroom with a singular purpose. It was time for my "lesson".

# 3

# FEAR

The interesting thing about fear is that it's a physical presence, as well as something much deeper. Throughout this book, as I open up about my past chapter by chapter, I want you to learn the process (emotional, cognitive, and physical) I had to go through in order to escape and overcome. For me, my body was in constant 'Survival Mode' when I was with my abuser. Anxiety filled me with each passing second. My fear and my responses not only affected me, but also fueled Her.

We all know what being afraid feels like; it's simple human nature. What may be less commonly understood, however, is that if we aren't careful, it can take over our mind and begin to control our actions. The brain has trouble processing anything outside of that emotion. And there are also different degrees of fear that any one person can experience at any given time. If we don't control our fear, it will control us. Fear is spiritual chaos.

The first key factor in overcoming this intense and unwelcome feeling is to both recognize it and address it. Stop and take a deep, slow breath, then take another. Breathing helps us stay connected with our body. The added oxygen in your brain helps your nervous system calm down. Your heart rate decreases, your breathing slows, and your mind is better able to process. It brings clarity for just a moment.

Next, ask the right questions in order to understand the fear. Where does it come from? Why am I fearful? What do I not yet know about myself that makes this fear bigger than it should be? What danger is fear warning me about? What needs to change to negate this fear? How is it affecting my daily life and relationships? Is this fear something that keeps me from reaching my potential? Sometimes shining light on the fear can reveal things about it that make it less threatening. Understanding can provide strength. It's okay to explore the fear.

Nowadays, the anxieties of my childhood do not hold power over me; I see them in a different light, but I still have fears. And I still use the same series of questions to process my fears and move forward. I do not let my fear make my decisions. I wish I had learned these lessons sooner, so I could have controlled my responses to my abuse.

When my abuser saw the fear in me, she honed in on it, and manipulated it. She twisted my thoughts in a way that convinced me I was helpless, that this was 'the way' things had to be. That I was weak. I was absolutely terrified of the woman, and this was something I had to overcome if I wanted to grow, to change for the better. Because it turns out, she was wrong about me. I wasn't weak. I just didn't know what I was capable of yet.

While I process my story with you, there is a key point

I must never overlook. All of my abuse occurred when I was only a child. Young. Alone. Scared. And fragile. But while I was only a young boy, there was already a hidden strength that would be revealed. Strength that was always inside of me, waiting to be found.

So, before I continue I want to say to you: YOU. ARE. STRONG. If you are going through something like what I experienced, I want to say: YOU. ARE. LOVED. This book in your hands is evidence. I'm writing my story for you. And if you feel like you have no purpose or that your life is meaningless, then I need you to hear me: YOU. ARE. SO. VALUABLE. Take these words I'm wanting you to hear and repeat them to yourself in the mirror. It'll take seconds of your life, but they are worth repeating. "I am strong. I am loved. I am valued." Words carry power, especially when coming from yourself.

You are resilient. And I understand the crippling fear that you may be feeling when you're alone or in a place you wish not to be. Inside of you is a strength that you must believe you have. Fear is useful. It is a natural tool that tells us things we need to know about how to survive, about what can protect us, but it is not what controls you. You control it.

Sometimes, fear sends you encrypted messages that only you would understand. Decrypt it in order to grasp what your mind and body are trying to tell you. Converse with it. Fear is an instinct to get you through the 'sucky' part of life. If fear is your inbuilt warning system — what danger is setting it off and what needs to change? Recognize and understand it, but never let it be your master.

You are going to get through this. You have to. The purpose and potential inside of you is just starting to grow. It's going to be hard. It's going to be a fight. But if you stand up and face that fear, if you are able to be patient with yourself and give yourself grace, then you will come out of this changed into someone ready to take on new and bigger things in this world. Strength is built through endurance. Endurance is repetition. Like when you work out, for example, your muscles get sore. In order to build up your muscles, you have to push past the discomfort.

We are all scared. We are all afraid. We all hurt in some way. Many of us feel like empty shells or disposed of. Each of us experience different levels of fear. The world has beat some of us down. Some of us want to give up. Don't. Stay in the fight. You have something to offer, even if you don't know what that is yet.

Own your fear. Learn from it. Overcome it. Again, this thing we call 'life' isn't very easy. When you get knocked down, get back up as soon as you can. It's not how you place, it's what you do with the result.

Take courage and stand strong. This world doesn't remember how many times you've fallen, only if you get back up.

Your courage defines your destiny.

# OVERTIME REFLECTION

- What are some things you fear?

- What obstacles have fear put in your life, and when do you notice fear the most?

- What is something you would do if you weren't afraid?

# 4

# CORPORAL PUNISHMENT

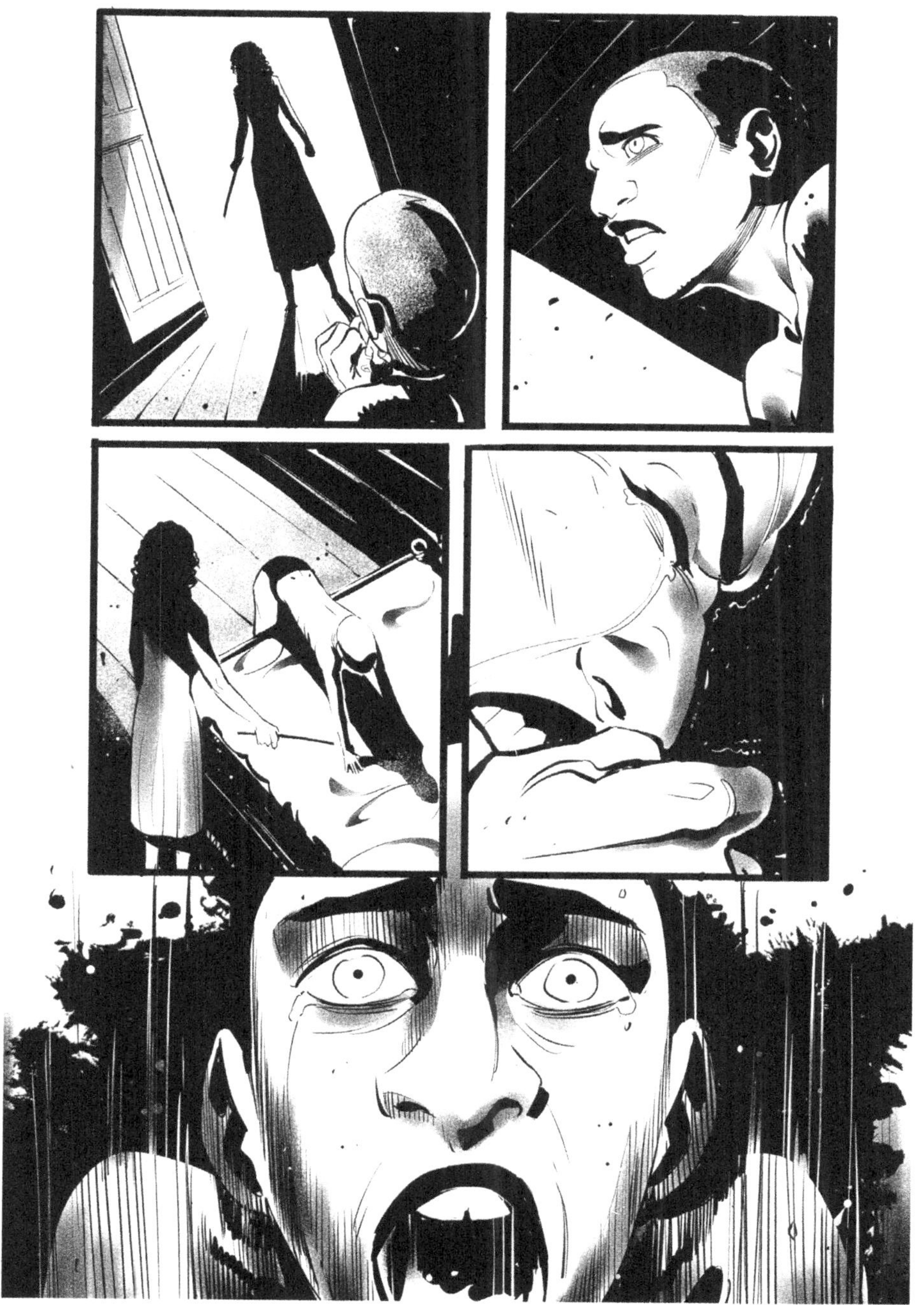

The doorway framed her dominating silhouette as the transparent glue stick refracted a tinge of fading moonlight from the window. That thing had been my nemesis since I was five years old; her weapon of choice for half a dozen years, and I was all too familiar with its bite. And before the dawn, I knew that I would feel it again.

Tears welled up in the corners of my eyes. I wasn't ready for this. I didn't want to be here. I longed to be teleported somewhere else. Anywhere else but here.

"Turn over," She demanded.

I knew what was coming and I couldn't stop the tears from flowing, just as I knew I wasn't going to be able to stop the beating. What could I possibly do to escape? Did she want me to beg? Fine, I could beg.

"Please, don't. I'm sorry. I'm sorry."

That made her madder. As if my words fell on deaf ears, she repeated coldly, "Turn over. Now."

Hesitantly, slowly, I rolled onto my stomach, futilely wishing my flesh to become indestructible. At the whoosh of the up-swing, I sucked in a deep breath, bracing for what was next. The millisecond felt endless, then CRACK! The glue-stick came down hard across my butt. The first initial hit was all it took for her dark side to erupt from its cocoon.

Another swing. And another.

WHOOSH CRACK WHOOSH CRACK WHOOSH CRACK

Up and down, the bludgeon cut the air. Like a conductor's baton, it directed the violent cadence of her raised voice, "DON'T. YOU. EVER.... "

Each snap hit harder than the last, the force of every strike sucking the breath out from my lungs. Within seconds, I was gasping for air, each breath cut short by the barrage from the force of the stick. My body curled into itself as if it had a mind of its own. Every muscle tight.

"I'm sorry!" I pleaded as tears poured down across my cheeks onto the blanket. My body was acting on its own will, and she didn't like that.

Oh, no she did not.

"ROLL OVER!"

"Please, no! I'm sorry!" Between us, my arms crossed over my body like a shield of protection.

"DO YOU WANT IT ON YOUR CHEST?" She bent down over me, a massive figure of apathetic anger. "OR ON YOUR BUTT?"

Slowly, she cocked her arm above her head, like the villain in a horror film, about to strike the fatal blow.

There was no escaping this. I was already in the deep end, and I was barely treading water. I felt like I was drowning, alone at the center of an ocean with only monsters of the deep beneath my feet.

I knew from experience that if I took the strikes to my chest, the wind would be knocked out of me. I didn't want to pass out, so I weighed my options and calculated the risks.

I submitted.

"On my butt," I whimpered.

"THEN ROLL OVER!"

Exposing my welted and swollen rear end, she started back up seemingly harder and louder than before. She was vengeful today, and I was nothing to her. Over and over, the terror endlessly descended.

"DON'T. YOU. EVER. HANG. UP. ON. ME!"

At this point, all I could really do was weep. There was nothing I could do or say to change her perception that I had hung up the school phone the day before without saying 'goodbye.'

# 5

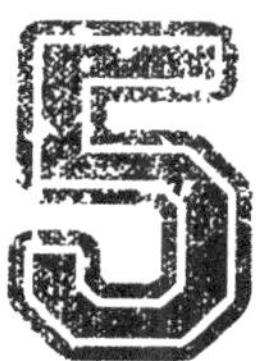

# SLEEVES AND A SMILE

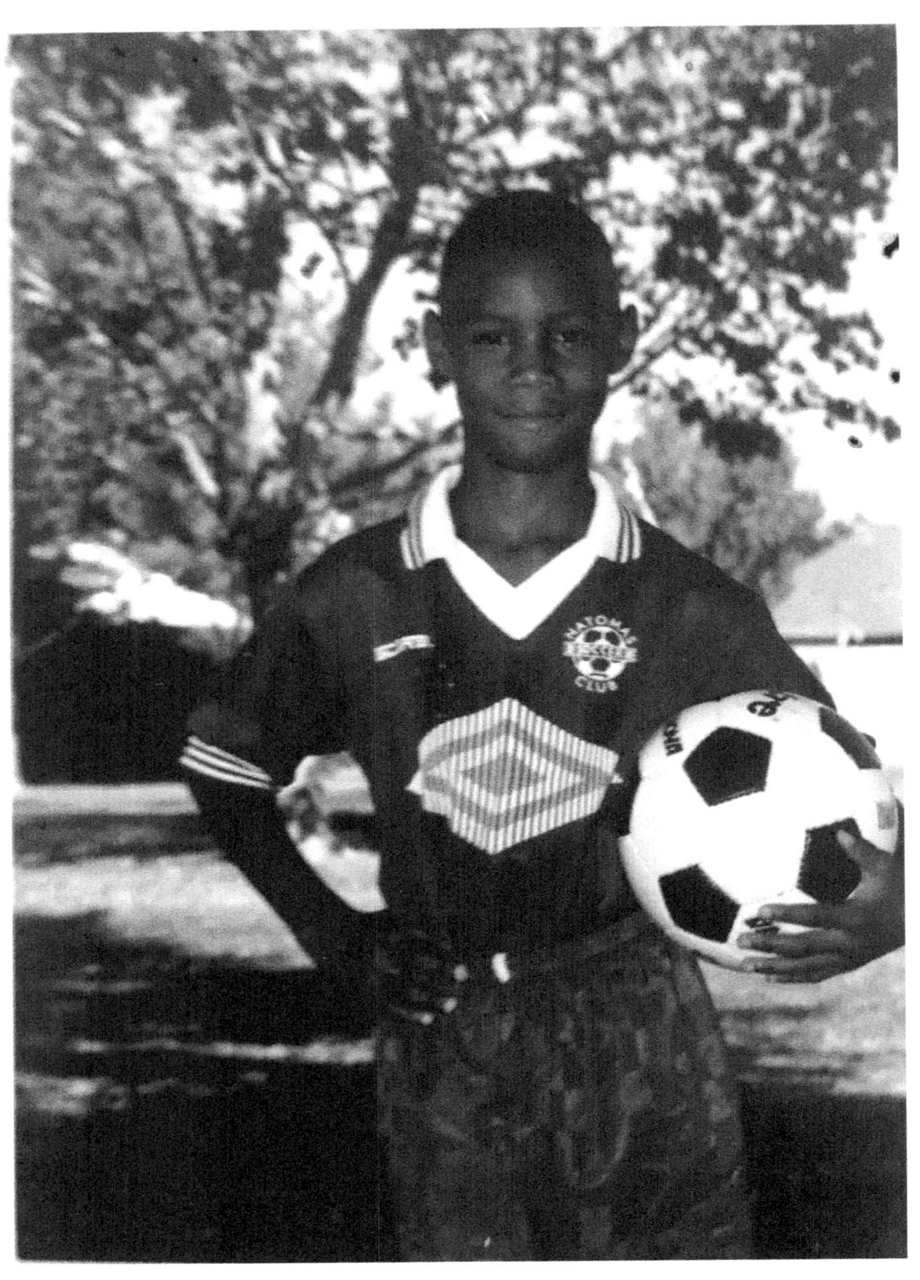

If someone from the future had come back in time to tell me that one day I would play in the NFL, I never would have believed them. No freakin' way. I would have laughed at them, called them 'crazy,' maybe even used a few choice words, and then told them to get lost.

Up to about seventh grade, I used to draw this epic cartoon called *The Rabbit vs V-1 Fighting Force*. Man, did I love it! I could become so engrossed in the story that it was an escape from the darkness I often endured. I had a safe place in my bedroom where I was able to isolate and just create in peace. Drawing gave me something to focus on, a better world to 'live in.'

Soccer was my game of choice. I was taller and stronger than most of my competitors. Also, playing soccer came naturally to me. I believed I had skills because I didn't have to work hard to be good at it. I would soon learn a valuable lesson that taught me otherwise. Sports hadn't fully become a passion yet and, despite my height, I didn't stand out for my athleticism. I wasn't picked first in recess. I wasn't someone everyone in my class wanted to be like. I just enjoyed playing.

Isaac Watt wrote a poem called 'False Greatness', stating:

*'Tis true, my form is something odd,*
*but blaming me, is blaming God;*
*Could I create myself anew*
*I would not fail in pleasing you.*

*If I could reach from pole to pole*
*or grasp the ocean with a span,*
*I would be measured by the soul;*

*The mind's the standard of the Man.*

I didn't yet know how to measure myself by the standard of my own mind. I was still looking outside of myself for those answers. I didn't know how to be me. I just did the sports scene because it was what my friends were doing. I had no real passion for it and I wasn't aware of what it could do to help me. I would have seized any opportunity that kept me away from my abuser a couple more hours a day. Like drawing, I used it to escape from my reality. If it took my mind off my personal pain, I was willing to try it.

One weekend when I was with my father, he took me to play basketball in a league he'd signed me up for. During one of the games, I was paired up against another kid. This kid was good. I mean, really good, and he just wrecked me. The whole game, up and down the court, he demonstrated what skill could do against whatever pride I *thought* I had from playing soccer.

Due to the emotional strain and physical abuse I endured as a child, my confidence was shot. I had none. How does a tween love himself when he is not treated lovingly by others? I didn't know how. I had extremely limited experience with actual love, so I was continually searching for it in every experience.

So I ended up crying on the bench. I couldn't handle it. The defeat devastated me. It felt like more evidence of a lack of love, and just added to all the low confidence I already had.

You see, I didn't have any sort of positive identity. I hated being who I was. I felt the world was against me, placing me in a life I didn't deserve. That's a lot of pain and confusion for a child to process. I didn't know which way to look for truth, so I was coming to my own conclusions and they weren't good ones. This made me bitter towards people who didn't know what I was going through, which was almost everyone.

I had every reason to be angry, confused, depressed, and lost. And most importantly, I felt absolutely alone — like a ghost in the crowd. All it took to hide my physical and emotional wounds were sleeves and a smile. No one was looking at the 'me' underneath.

So how did I handle everything? I hid my 'mess of a childhood' with a smile for my friends and cold shoulders for the rest, especially the adults. I put on an act to show I wasn't weak. I was intimidated by adults and the power they could wield. I did my best to simply disappear into the background.

Maybe you know what it means to try to 'blend in.' That's not something to feel ashamed about. We do what we must to make it to the next day, but as I have said before — and I will reiterate throughout this book — you are not alone.

The world is full of bullies, but it is also full of heroes. There are *numerous* people who have spent many, many years improving their craft as human service workers — counselors, mentors, life coaches, doctors, therapists, coaches, social service workers … the list goes on. Sometimes, it's not even someone who has dedicated their life to helping people, but just someone who feels a connection to *you*. There are people out there who can help you. They *want* to help you. Find these heroes. Let them find you.

Remember the story above, where I was distraught and defeated, sitting on the bench? Well, let me continue with what happened afterward. My father saw me crying and understood something I didn't yet. Together we left and drove through the dark to a nearby high school where there was an outdoor basketball court lit up by streetlights.

He parked the car, then turned to me and said, "'If you want to be great, then you'll meet me at the free throw line. And if you're not out there when I get to the free throw line, then I'll come back to the car and we'll never say another word about it."

He got out of the car and started walking. I didn't know what to do. This was a choice, an opportunity to change, and even though I didn't understand yet, I trusted him. I got out of the car and ran to the court. I made it to the free throw line, and then he said something I'll never forget. "That kid wasn't better than you. He just put more work in than you."

I started crying on the spot as he walked to me and gave me a hug. That single, *true* statement planted a seed deep in my spirit. From that point on, I had a passion to sprout that seed and see what it could become. The more I continued to take his words to heart and *try*, the bigger it grew! I could have easily disregarded his advice. I could have let my pain make my decisions or close me off to someone who truly cared about me. I could have ignored the support and encouragement. But I didn't, and it made all the difference in my life. I allowed him to care for me and offer his wisdom. When wisdom is offered to you, let it all soak in. Your seed needs that water to grow.

You may not have a person like I did who is part of your family or close circle, but there are many others out there who have wisdom to offer. When you're ready, I encourage you to reach out to those helpers and professionals and teachers and counselors. They have experience with 'life.' Don't try to take this world on by yourself. Human beings are tribal, we're a community. We were not designed to go through our entire lives alone. Teachers need students and vice versa. Coaches need athletes and vice versa. Doctors need patients and vice versa. The world is a big place where you can lose yourself, so find someone who can help guide you down the path of success instead of failure. I don't want you lost. I want you found.

The deeper you look into your own heart, the deeper you'll start looking into the hearts of the people around you. The more you seek out your own potential and gifts, the easier it will be for you to see others'. Before long, you'll be able to see past the sleeve and smiles, to their hearts. This is what it's like to love another human, to see their greatness inside of them. But you must recognize the greatness inside of you first. Instead of hiding, start soul-searching and discovering who you are. You are somebody special.

And to the helpers of the world who may also be

reading this, give people hope by telling them you believe in them, even when they don't believe in themselves. Because once you plant those seeds hope will grow inside them like a wild vine. And the more you keep showing up in their lives, day after day and month after month and year after year, the stronger they will grow. Words have the power to give life. Speak truth and inspiration every day. Encourage them. Help them heal. Tend to their spirit and passions.

Doubt is infectious, but love is even more so.

For me, through years of hiding my pain, I was scared to be vulnerable. I blended in as someone else instead of sharing who I really was. And that's only because of fear. Fear of what other people would think of me. Relationships with other kids were shallow. I chose to play 'life' as someone else. Whoever I truly was at the time was hidden in a shadow of different identities, different personas.

Now, not all of us handle our struggles in the same way. And we all deal with unique circumstances. I chose hiding in order to survive. Others may tend to lean into vices that provide distractions, but cause their own range of problems. Some of us find the crowd who make us feel good (whether or not they actually *are* good), who help us forget the crap we have experienced. Others find a variety of healthy or unhealthy means to cope. We respond to fear, pain, and anger in so many different ways. But it doesn't make you any *less* of a human ... just human.

Many people may not be aware, but for some of us survival is like a subchapter to our life story, a different journey or path that runs parallel to all those other 'regular' lives. We don't yet know where life will take us once we break through the struggle. It can feel like we are trudging through the weeds in the ditch, while the rest of the world walks freely on the open road. Just keep moving forward and there will be a day when the way will begin to clear before you. Keep your eyes looking forward, where you will find your true path.

Now, for those individuals who are like me — *were* like me — just continue to recognize and process the fears and pain. We all have messy stuff about our lives — now, back then, or even coming soon. The longer you hide the mess, the more it will pile up and threaten to fall out of the closet on you. Eventually you can't hold it all back and your mess will be exposed.

It's okay to hurt and hide and struggle and fall. I've been there. I'm encouraging you not to give up on yourself. Those obstacles created strength in me that never would have been there otherwise. Take heart! You contain greatness! It grows inside of you even now. People are cheering for you, whether you realize it or not. They may be people struggling just like you, waiting for your strength and courage to become a pillar for them to lean on. Don't give up on them. Don't give up on yourself.

Sooner or later, we are all found. This is a good thing. We all want to be rescued from the dark, but sometimes we hide in it because we're familiar with it, because it feels safer. But it's not.

Step out into the light.

# OVERTIME REFLECTION

- What parts of your identity do you hide from others?

- Why do you feel the need to hide those parts?

- Who would you be if you could just be yourself?

# 6

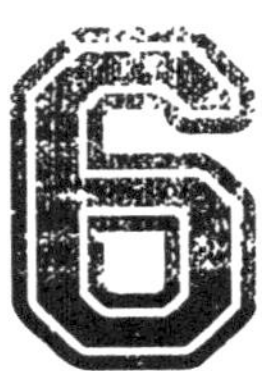

# ACTIONS ARE LOUDER THAN WORDS

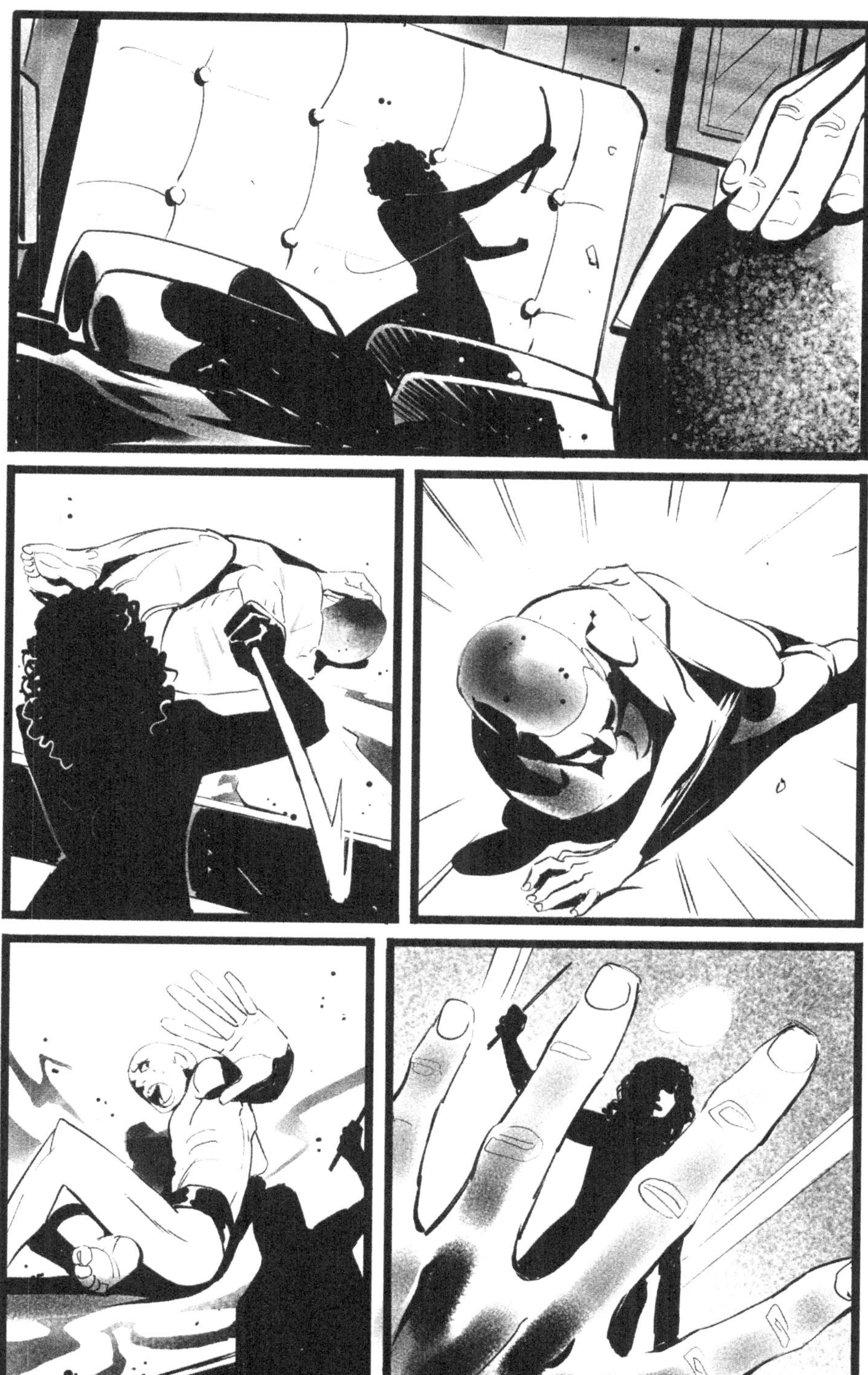

The beating was endless. As if my wailing wasn't distressed enough for her, she moved from my butt to my thighs; a fresh place to continue her rain of fury. I didn't know how long it had been going on, but it was chaos; chaos in my mind and in my body. Together, she and I were stuck in this moment that seemed to last forever. It felt as though the rest of the world had frozen. Only her tireless arm remained in motion, moving up and down, over and over my bruised and battered body. This nightmare was terrifying. I just wanted to wake up.

I don't even know when *exactly* the yelling had stopped. The verbal 'lesson' had apparently ended, but she was far from finished with teaching me something. What was it? It didn't matter. She probably didn't even know herself. She was lost in her own haze of pain and sorrow and wrath.

The world was muted, and the only sound in the room was the impact of the glue stick and my cries. I never knew if the neighbor heard anything, but I'm sure my crying was loud enough.

I wasn't a small kid either. At eleven years old, I was already around 5'8" and 140 pounds, close to her size, physically, but that didn't matter to her. I was still small in her eyes.

I couldn't help the 'why me' questions that arose. Why me, someone who was begging for all this to stop? Why me, someone who was supposed to be protected by her? Why me, someone who was a good kid? These were the wrong questions. They didn't matter.

Once again, I rolled over and attempted to shield myself. I don't know where I found the courage, but for the first time I opened my eyes and actually looked at her. Her actions became an instant recording in my mind as I took in the sweat of her exertion and the blinding fury on her face. I could see her heavy breathing widening her nostrils as her chest and shoulders heaved. And I could see the pain in her eyes. Her own pain.

I willed her to see me, to see what she was doing to me. I wanted her to know I existed in this moment with her, but the expression on her face was empty of anything but rage, like a distorted Halloween mask.

In my squirming attempt to shield myself with flailing limbs, her weapon found more fresh, exposed areas of my body that my arms weren't protecting. *WHACK!!* Readjust, *WHACK!!* Over and over again. It was like a sick game of whack-a-mole. With her arm raised, she'd aim, wait, then re-engage.

The fight appeared futile, but for some reason, I wouldn't allow myself to fully give up or give in. I pulled from a deep, inner reserve of strength and made the conscious decision to protect myself emotionally, by any means necessary. I had to. I didn't know when (or if) she was going to stop. I didn't know if my body was going to survive, but I decided, in that moment, that my mind *would*.

The barrage triggered numbness in certain places on my body, which meant my brain's defense mechanisms were beginning to kick in. The clear hiss of the stick continued to cut through the air, punctuated by the continual *crack* on my skin like a firecracker.

A few clean shots to the legs forced me to curl up tightly. The pain was overwhelming. The only breaths I could muster when they weren't knocked out of me were spent on my sobs. The fear remained.

As the onslaught kept up, however, something occurred to me. Something woke up inside of my thoughts. The physical pain didn't matter anymore. It really didn't. That pain was becoming secondary to the true pain I was feeling.

No. You see, what mattered the most was not what She was doing to me, but the fact that she was doing it at all.

Suddenly, I knew I couldn't allow this to happen any longer.

# 7

# TIME SEES YOUR WORTH

The lesson I learned that morning was not the 'lesson' my abuser was teaching me. It was something much bigger. To be honest, that moment reshaped my whole perspective on life entirely. A new awareness awoke in me and somehow revealed all the different avenues of my life, all the possibilities.

Was it good she did this to me? ABSOLUTELY NOT! It never should have happened. But it did, and somehow that caused a shift in me. It brought truth to my life.

Living in survival mode, I was always on alert. My radar was always on for her escalations, body language, warnings, red flags — when I was around her. Whenever I was with my friends or other people, it was always a heavenly, peaceful time for me. I didn't have to 'survive' in these settings. I could think about video games, watching TV, eating junk food, and not having to worry about my homework.

But there were instances that pushed me to mature quicker. When I was with my dad, I acted older than I was, yet when I was in my abuser's house, I acted younger than I was. I played innocent, childish, needy.

My brain was forced to mature faster than most kids. I had to think about things differently than other kids. My priorities were different when I was in the place that was unsafe for me. And because I wasn't allowed to behave and act like an ordinary kid, I saw my life in an unhealthy way.

But after this pivotal moment with my abuser and the glue stick, I became aware of my existence, and while I still lay weeping on the bed, I didn't want to be erased from the world. I realized that my life was precious. Invaluable. And extremely fragile.

While all these things occurred, 99.99999% of the world didn't know who I was or what I was going through. But over the years, many came to know it, and now you know it too. And it matters. Not just for myself, but for every single one of you who needs to know your value. This is part of my platform and purpose. Everyday life is intrinsically important. Every hour, every minute are like tiny gifts from the future given to us on an assembly line. Moments in time that we didn't know we'd get. And I realize that every decision we make can shape and reshape our future — for good or bad. Reach for the right pieces and you will build something beautiful.

We take time for granted. We waste it. We just want to get by or make time go faster or wait until tomorrow. Why?! What has made *this* moment less valuable than the next? The 'now' is where we construct our future. Shaping our future is how we learn from our past.

Time is something we don't fully appreciate until it

has already passed us by. As we get older and reflect on our past, most people feel regret for not appreciating the value of their time or not using it wisely. How many millions of people didn't get to work the career they were meant to work? How many people didn't fulfill their dreams and hopes and aspirations? How many people felt 'later' was like the greener grass on the other side of the fence?

To be honest, I never thought I'd live to be a teenager, let alone a grown man. Yet, here I am. With you. Telling you that time doesn't stop moving, so take ahold of it and make it everything it's meant to be.

Even when I'm long gone from this world, the impact of my time here can continue.  Like a pebble thrown in a lake, the ripples continue after the stone disappears from the surface. I'm going to spend my time telling you how incredibly valuable you are. But in your life, you need to find your place, your purpose, your destiny. You have no idea where that ripple will go. Once you overcome your fear, seek out the reason you were put on this planet and how to make your life something good.

There are so many others like us who have known struggle and fear and pain and despair and haven't found the courage to step out into their own purpose. So let's stand tall for them. Let them see the path they can also walk. Be a part of something with that greatness inside of you. See yourself as a chest full of treasure. What value does it have buried on a private island? Treasure only matters when it's found and shared. Your greatness is meant to be shared with the world, not buried and hidden. Even if that world is just one person, it still matters.

Most of all, stand strong for you. You are worthy of this life. You are worthy of the gifts that Time offers. You exist and you're capable of greatness. Just believe it. To believe in yourself is to know that you aren't a waste.

Let me encourage you also, Time will probably throw you curveballs; maybe something you didn't think would come your way. It could be another obstacle. It could be another trial. It could be another temptation or another moment of failure. But failure teaches us as many great lessons as we let it.

Time is also just as likely to bring about opportunities. A second chance. An open door. A new path, and even more lessons to grow from. And the best thing about Time: it doesn't give you an opportunity too big for you to handle. It's a gradual gift-giver that builds on itself. It wants you to succeed. I want you to succeed.

You see, my life belongs to me. It always did. Not Her, not to anyone else. And it was in this moment of seeming defeat that I somehow saw myself in a different light. The abuse had preyed upon me for six years, and I could no longer depend on others to stand up for me. I had to take that first stand on my own, with my own new-found strength. It wasn't going to be easy. But once I made the choice, then I knew Time would put more people in my life who could believe in me, who could support me.

But do you know why I did it, why I had to stand up for myself? Well, that's the right question.

Because I'm worthy of my life, just like you are. And I have time to make it worthwhile.

## OVERTIME REFLECTION

- What traumatic experience has you stuck in the past?

- What pieces do you want to let go of?

- How do you see yourself in the present moment, and is this where you want to be?

# 8

# IT'S OVER WHEN SHE SAYS IT IS

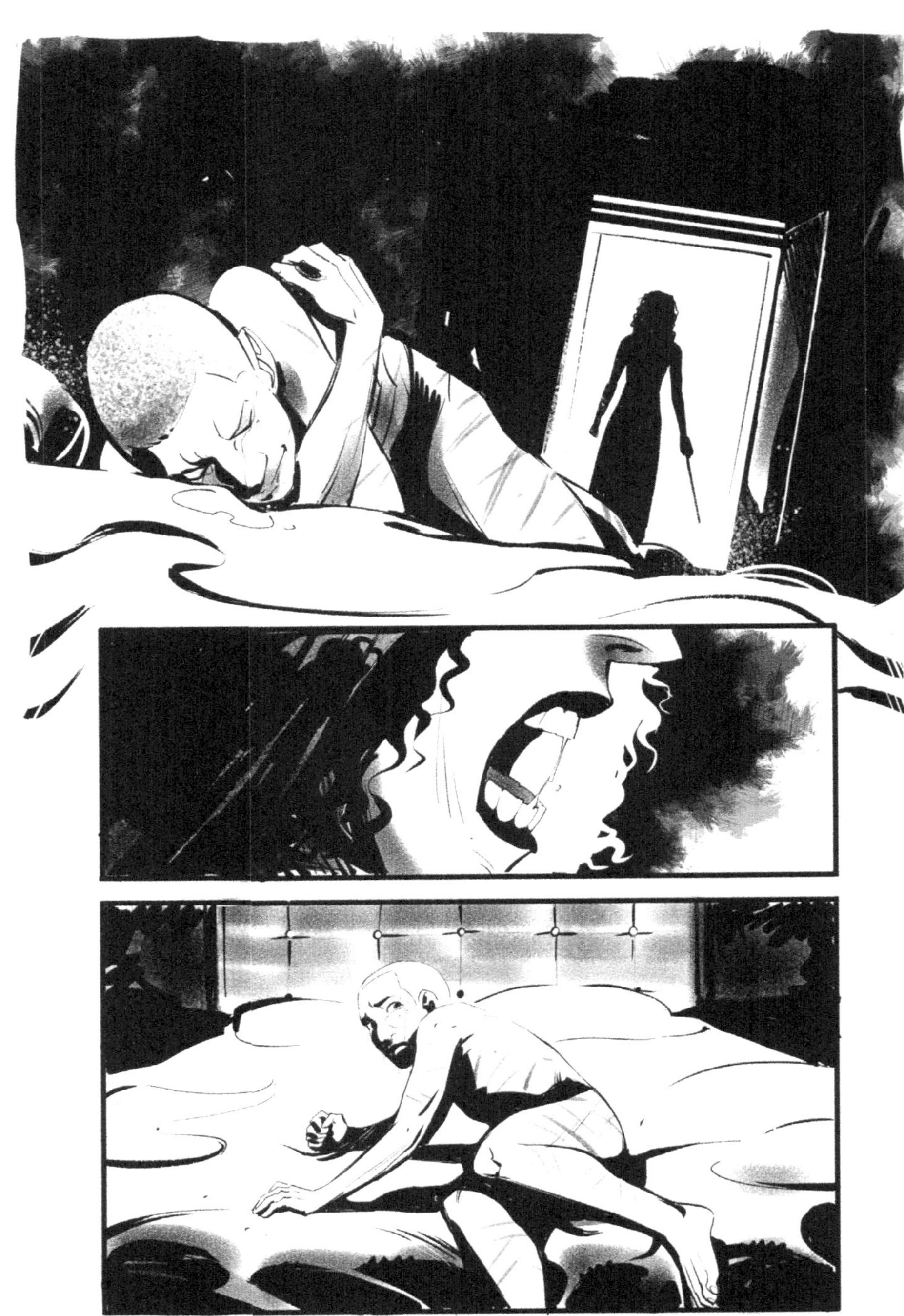

Just as suddenly as it had begun, the beating stopped.

Over the quiet sound of my dejected sobs and rasping breath, I could hear her voice speaking coldly, "You will never disrespect me like that again, do you hear me? … DO. YOU. HEAR. ME?"

She had finally concluded her 'lesson,' now all she needed was confirmation that her point had been made.

"DO YOU HEAR ME?!" she repeated. She loomed over me, waiting for an answer.

Breathing was still hard, but I managed to croak out a quiet, "Yes."

I think it made her uncomfortable to see me in such a broken state, knowing what she had just done to me. Any human with a soul has the ability to see the error of their ways if they actually look, but by this point, there was no changing what she had just put me through. Did I expect an apology… no. I was just glad it was over.

"Now, go take a shower." She exhaled hard and turned for the door. "We are going to go to church." And just like that, she was gone.

Strangely, there was still a part of me that hoped she would come back into the room and apologize and tell me everything was going to be alright; that this was never going to happen again. Somehow I still knew I deserved to be shown love, but that wasn't her style, so I pushed the empty hope aside, focusing instead on what was next, church. I know for some of you reading this, hearing about a "church" woman beating the living hellfire out of me may sound overwhelmingly hypocritical, and you'd be right. It was a complete contradiction in itself, but to me, the idea of church was a breath of heaven! Going to Church meant being in public, one of the safest places for me, even if just for a few hours.

When my abuser was around church folks, she was an angel. She was everything I needed in my life when others were around. Of course, I knew it was just a facade. She hid the 'real' person very well, and only I knew the darkness she carried inside. She blended in, just like I did at school. Wearing church clothes and a smile. She didn't want anyone else to know what really existed in the depths of her soul, and I honestly don't blame her. Nobody wants people to know the bad things they have done behind closed doors. So if she was going to be an angel, well ... it was what I needed and I wasn't going to stop her.

From my place on the bed, I heard her return the glue stick to its drawer, until next time, then continued about her business as if nothing had ever happened.

Alone with my pain, I wondered how much longer my

life was going to be like this, and how much more of this I was going to be able to take. My biggest fear was that this would last forever, or that one day these beatings would beat the life out of me.

As the pain started to subside some, I could begin processing my thoughts more clearly. My brain was still hazy and overstimulated, but I remembered what I was supposed to do, and gingerly scooched to the end of the bed with my arms little by little, trying not to use my legs too much. Getting to my feet, my body felt too heavy for my battered legs. Step by agonizing step, I trudged weakly to the bathroom, closed the door, and locked it. That little click made my whole world feel just a little bit safer. This wooden door was my wall of protection from what lay on the other side of it.

Hesitantly, slowly, I turned around and looked in the mirror. I didn't recognize the person looking back at me. Gasping and trying not to cry, I simply stared.

# 9

# FINDING THE BRIGHT SPOT

There is power in positive thinking, but in my situation as a child, I would have disagreed. I would have said that positivity was for people who knew nothing about real hardship. I would have blown up on someone who told me to be positive, or completely written them off.

But over time, I came to find out how true it was. My brain wielded much more power than I knew. But first, there had to be an attitude change, a new philosophy to my existence. Basically I needed a shift in how I viewed myself and my role in this world. It was not an easy thing to do, because I had very little emotional resilience to care about things — or people. I hated my life, but there came a point where I needed to change the way I was thinking. The more I thought hatefully, the more my perspective on life and people distorted into a hateful mindset towards nearly everything.

The way I started to change, began with focusing on anything outside of the house — places that weren't in the darkness. Let's just call these places my bright spots. These were the places or people or things where the darkness of my life couldn't exist. These places lit up the dark corners of my soul. I was able to think differently, behave differently, and live differently. And differently was a good thing.

Whenever I was able to see my dad, things were pretty structured. He always had something special for us to do or he'd let me just chill as I played Dreamcast or the Playstation. But there came a point when he started teaching me things here and there as well.

I remember, one time we were heading to the grocery store. Seemingly out of nowhere, he announced, "Hey, this is going to be a different weekend. Before you play video games, you have to memorize this poem." He handed me a sheet of paper. I didn't even bother looking at it. I just responded exactly like most kids would — complain and object to the idea.

He responded simply, "Well, it's going to be a quiet weekend, then."

The poem he wanted me to memorize was called "Invictus," written by William Ernest Henley when he was dying from Tuberculosis. I was a determined kid, and I really wanted to play my video games, so instead of pouting or staying in the car while he went shopping, I ran in with him. As we shopped together, my dad had me read the lines aloud, repeating them over and over. By the time we were ready to check out, I had the entire poem memorized. He told me to keep practicing it even when I wasn't staying with him. This poem was deep and each line was a treasure trove of wisdom. I'll share more about my love of poetry in a later chapter.

For the most part, the adults either treated me well or ignored me. I was one of the masses. I knew what to expect at school, and I could learn and participate in things that were enjoyable.

Sometimes kids who have gone through what I did, use the school environment as their bright spot. I certainly did. School for me was a place that was structured. My friends were there. There was one friend in particular, who we'll call Ray. We had been friends since kindergarten, and he was one of those bright spots I could go to. For years, I shared with him stories about my ongoing abuse. I knew I could trust him with this secret; and the pain I was all too often experiencing. At some point in our friendship, something prompted him to wisely break our confidence and share with his mother what was going on. I didn't learn this until much later, but his mother took this information very seriously and also made the right choice. She told my father. This would prove to be very helpful to my safety and well-being later down the road.

In the meantime, sports, crushing on girls, free food, laughter, gossip, and even staring out windows in class meant the world to me. All these things filled me with a little bit of happiness and relief. These were little gems — bright spots — that I could focus on throughout the day.

But school is not a place of escape for everyone. And I want you to know I understand that, too. For many of you, you feel you can't succeed emotionally or socially at school either. The anxieties and trauma of life and abuse you may be experiencing within those walls can be crippling. School may even feel like a worse place than home.

I'm still going to encourage you to find the bright spots. Find people who can be pillars for you, and it may mean getting out of your comfort zone to meet kids different from you. Or speak to trustworthy adults you don't know yet. If they smile and want to know your passions and hobbies, then connect. Steer clear of people whose influence will take you down a path that leads away from your dreams and hopes. Get to know a teacher or counselor who seems to care about you, because I am certain they truly do. Sincerity is so important to have in your life. As I've mentioned before, let yourself be found. You may not be able to see all the bright spots yet, but many people around you already have "flashlights" that they know how to use. Let them shine some light in the darkness. Let them share their light with you as you seek out your own.

I want you to know that you've got this. Don't let every place you go be made of darkness and fear. Take it one day at a time, and push yourself through it. Ask for help from people you can lean on. I want you to succeed, and I want you to feel peace and purpose wherever you can, so find it in places that help you grow and love yourself, not corrode you from the inside out.

If you are battling every day for your life, just know that you are loved. You are strong. Stronger than you think yourself to be. Believe I am thinking about you as I work on this book, hoping it becomes one of your bright spots. My heart goes out to you, and if this book has found you, just know that I have found you.

Now, let's focus on our mindset. The mind is an extremely powerful tool. When ingrained deeply enough, ideas and thoughts become core beliefs, the foundation that everything else is built on. Some of those thoughts can be contagious and can impact people they come in contact with — of course, I'm talking about both ends of the spectrum, good and bad. They have power!

When I was a child, my mindset was focused on getting to those bright spots as much as possible, like the poetry I mentioned earlier. The lines of poetry I memorized had the ability to ground me when I felt lost, hurt, or alone.

You see, my life was pretty dark. I'm only telling you one piece of the story, but there was so much more that I had already experienced leading up to this moment. If I took the time to write it all out, this book would probably be the size of an encyclopedia. So within that darkness,

I was desperate for light, for love, and for goodness. But with friends, poetry, drawing, and sports, I had a little bit of hope; and that was another bright spot because hope shines an incredibly potent light.

When I found light, I held on to it. I would do everything in my power to keep it, even if it was just for a short time. When I was in the home of my abuser, walking on eggshells, I couldn't wait until I found my next bright spot. It was the only thing I had to look forward to, and sometimes it wouldn't come for days or weeks — like getting to see my dad again.

School was one of those bright spots, as was church and even other family member's homes. These were the places I had the best chances of being a kid. I took advantage of it. I joined sports, church plays, and clubs as much as I could. Bright spots allowed me to push all the mess into the back of my mind.

There are so many of us out there who know what it means to live in a dark place — heavy, uncertain, cold, unanchored, lonely, and full of terror. Don't sit in that darkness with nothing good in your mind or heart.

While it is true that the world is full of darkness and evil, and often things don't make sense and distort how we see ourselves. It is also true that there are bright spots all around as well, where we can make sense of things, see the good the world has to offer, and view ourselves in a whole new light. Whatever good you put in your life can change how you see yourself in this big Earth.

Find the bright spots. And when you find them, engage in them. Sit in them and soak up the light. Reflect on your future and your strengths. Keep your mindset positive, and soon not only will it provide you courage in the darkness, but you will become a bright spot for others.

## OVERTIME REFLECTION

- What are some of the bright spots in your life?

- When was a time that you needed a bright spot in your life?

- Are your bright spots healthy and safe for your mind and body?

# 10

# BRUISED AND BEATEN

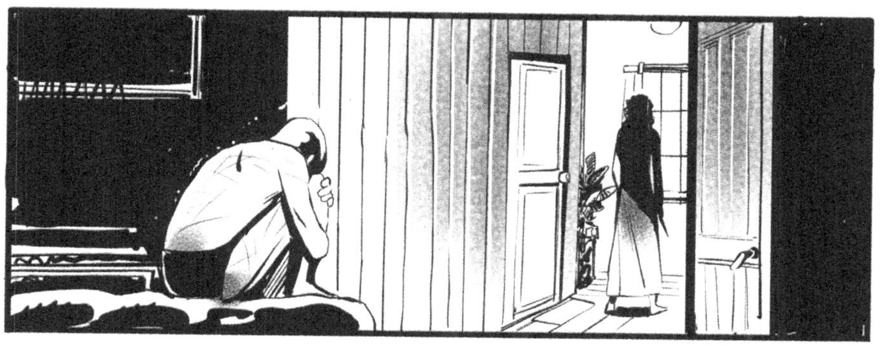

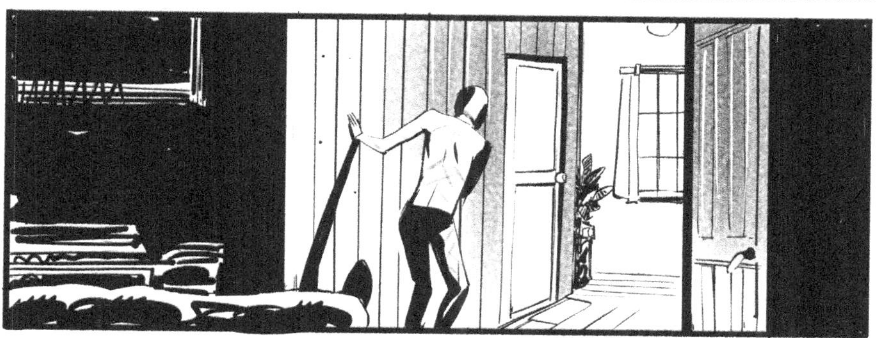

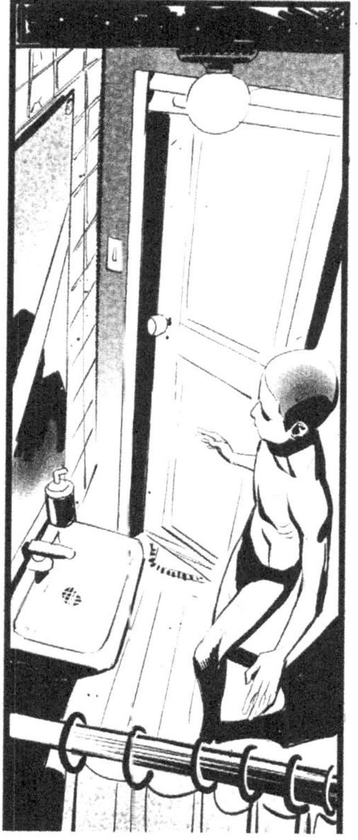

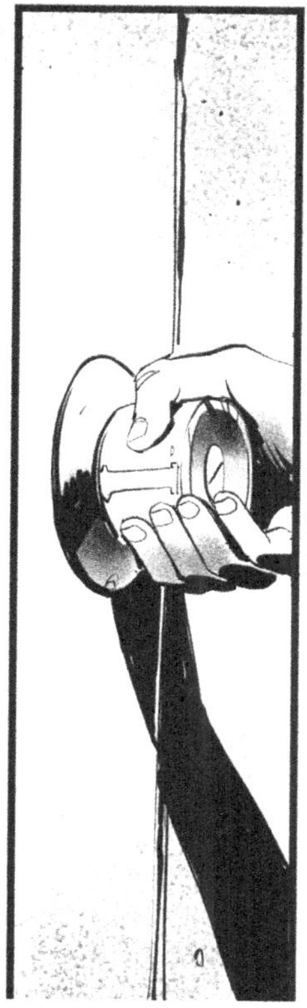

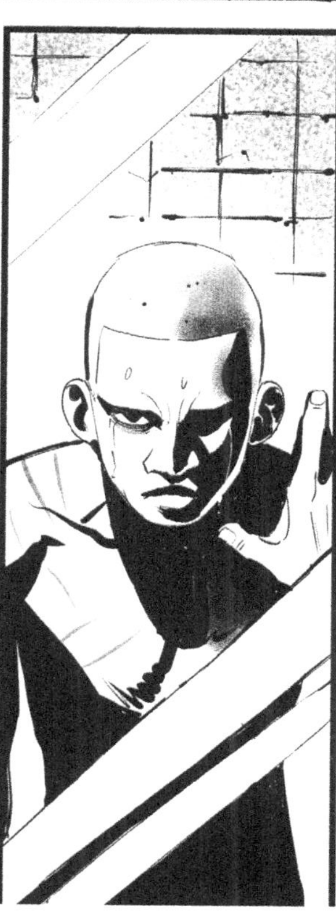

I couldn't stop shaking. Not because I was cold and nearly naked, but because my body had gone through such an intense moment of abuse that it was trying to readjust to the pain. My brain was processing the damage, just as I was. I was in absolute agony. What was a boy to think after something like this? How long was I willing to endure this life and this constant state of fear and pain? Why did I deserve this? Was I a bad person?

Fresh tears streamed down my cheeks as I took in the reflection in the mirror and felt the pain of my battered emotions. There was shame in the eyes looking back at me, shame that this had happened to me. I didn't want to see, but I couldn't look away. My body was riddled with welts, cracked skin, and bruises. Some areas were much worse than others. I barely recognized my grotesquely swollen body. It was like a bad reaction to a food allergy. And everything just hurt.

I stripped off my underwear to get a full view of the damage. An eleven-year-old boy, naked and afraid, I longed to stay in the shelter of this bathroom forever. I knew my red eyes, swollen from crying would quickly fade, but the damage on my body would not be so quick to heal. Would these bruises be gone before the next 'lesson'? Was this what life was supposed to be like for me? Was I so weak that I wouldn't survive? Did I even want to?

As much as I had hoped and prayed, my skin was not made of armor after all. I counted over fifteen major welts, and those were just the ones I could see, just the ones that radiated the most pain. One welt, behind my right knee, was particularly painful. Putting weight on it was even worse. I had never seen one so big before. It was grossly inflamed and hot to the touch. Everything just hurt, and each time I found a new injury, a shock of pain went through me, replaying the beating in my mind like a highlight reel.

As usual, she had been smart enough to only strike me where a long sleeve shirt and pants would cover. Had she hit me in the face, we wouldn't have been able to go to church that day. Thankfully, she hadn't. I needed to be around church folks right now.

As I assessed my body, I began to feel a sense of anger. Was this going to be the rest of my life? My abuser was someone who was supposed to love me, but this was not love. I knew what love felt like. The longer I resided in the anger, the more it began to evolve into hate.

At that very moment, however, my father's faithful efforts to teach me poetry came into play. The sorrowful words of William Ernest Henley's poem "Invictus" sprang from my distorted thoughts and realigned my spirit within me.

*Under the bludgeonings of chance,*
*my head is bloodied but unbowed.*

Then a still, quiet voice inside said something I would never forget. Words that would replay in my head over and over again.

*"When I am bigger than her, she won't be able to do this anymore. I won't allow it."*

# 11

# DON'T GIVE UP. GET UP

Maya Angelou once said, "You will face many defeats in life, but never let yourself be defeated." And how true her words are. My young, frail self felt defeated every single day. That moment, locked in the bathroom, is ingrained in my memory to this day. And that's okay. Some scars remain for a purpose. I can look at a scar as a reason to still feel angry or hurt, or I can look at it as a reminder that I have a story to tell. Either way, it's a part of me forever. And I'm no longer scared to show it. You know why?

That's the right question. Because attitude is everything. The definition of "attitude" is more or less your settled way of thinking about something that is reflected in your behavior; the way you think affects your actions.

As those tears ran down my eleven-year-old face, clarity had finally hit me — clarity of my existence. I realized I was a person, a human being. I wasn't some puppet. She couldn't attempt to destroy me anymore.

Reflected in the mirror was a boy who hadn't had a chance at life yet. I was full of darkness, anger, confusion, and resentment. But I suddenly understood that giving up wasn't the way to go. It was time for me to make my stand. I needed to be better, just like my father had challenged me to be on the basketball court. If I wanted to be better, then

I needed to step up to that free throw line and push myself.

The kid in the mirror was an innocent victim. He wasn't a bad kid. Just lost and alone. And I loved him. I was just starting to see that. And this was the point in my story where that little seed of courage had finally sprouted from within the darkness inside of me, and I knew I had to take a stand against Her. Not because she was my enemy, but because she was not going to decide my life. I needed to take charge and be accountable for me and what was happening to me.

So how did I do it? That's the right question. By this point, I wanted to live so badly that my mind began to search for the bright spots I somehow knew would bring me hope. I began to mentally strategize. And that's what I encourage you to do also. Find your hope.

Don't *give* up. **Get up!** Get up and search for those good things, no matter how few or small they may be.

I had realized that if *I* wanted change, then I needed to change. I couldn't wait on my abuser to change, and I couldn't wait for others to notice my struggles before coming to the rescue. No. It was I who had to change. It needed to start with me.

In that moment, my philosophy about myself changed. I began to think differently. I began to understand how I could adapt and grow stronger in those environments. And once I found that support within myself, my heart began to change.

I realized that I needed to find a 'someone' to reveal my secret to. Up to this point, I hadn't really had help, but I knew that if I wanted to get through this, I had to find a person to help me. A bright spot. Someone who could take a stand alongside me. And I did.

When you are able to find someplace or someone that provides just a little bit of safety, new emotions may arise that are hard to process. I found for myself, places of safety triggered overwhelming confusion. It took me a long time to learn how to control my anxiety and trauma response. It's okay if this happens to you, too. Stay with the feelings and the safe people and places, and let them help you in this process. Reorganizing your emotional world back into the order that will best serve your needs isn't easy, but it will be life-changing. You have a lot of learning to do, so be patient with yourself. You are worth it!

Struggle is hard, but it's so much easier to go through when you are able to find those special people to lean on. If you let others invest in you, if you let others help carry the burden with you, then the climb up and out of the valley will create momentum up the mountain. Don't run from the struggle. Fight through it. Grow through it.

Find that supportive coach, that inspiring teacher,

that genuine counselor, that uplifting neighbor — people that see the good in you. These are the ones who want the best for you, who see the greatness in you, who know that you exist. They may say 'hi' to you in the hallway or throw an arm around your shoulders at church. These certain special people may even open up to you first. People don't have to be blood to understand your pain. They are the ones who want to know you're happy, and they'll do what they can in order to help you through that struggle.

Don't reach out to anyone who puts you down, or makes you feel the way your abuser does. Go to the ones who are speaking love and truth and life, even if it's hard truths. And don't make them do all the work. They can't make your choices for you, but they can be loving guides. Do what you can to make the most of their love.

Don't give up, get up. Trust in yourself and take a stand.

# OVERTIME REFLECTION

- How do you react when things don't go your way?

- What is keeping you from growing, and what excuses are holding you back?

- What's your attitude towards life, and are you your own barrier?

# 12

# REACHING FOR A BRIGHT SPOT

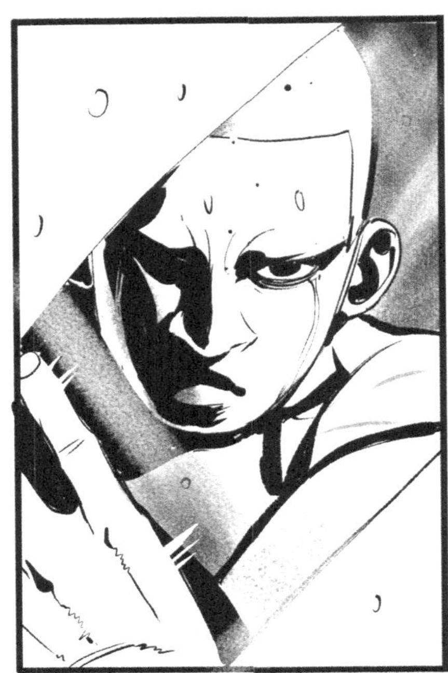
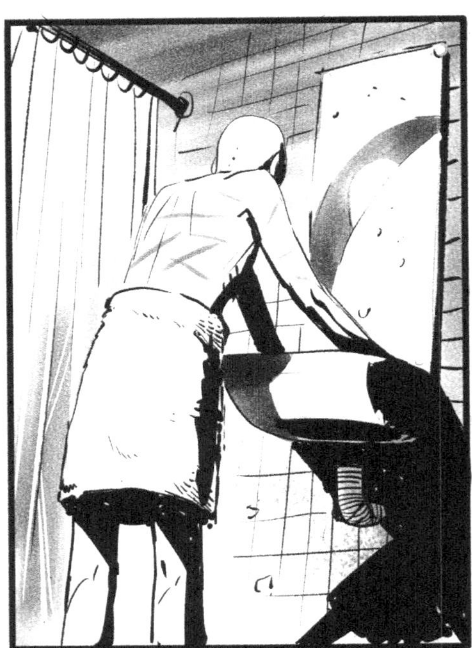
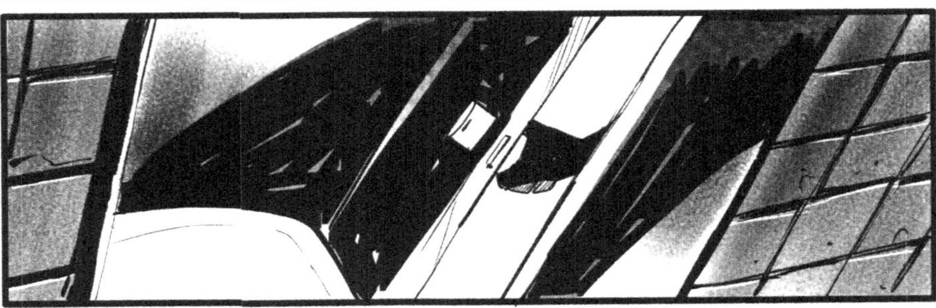
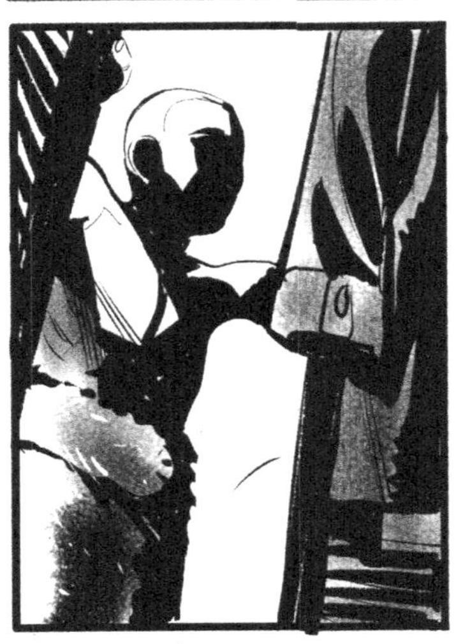
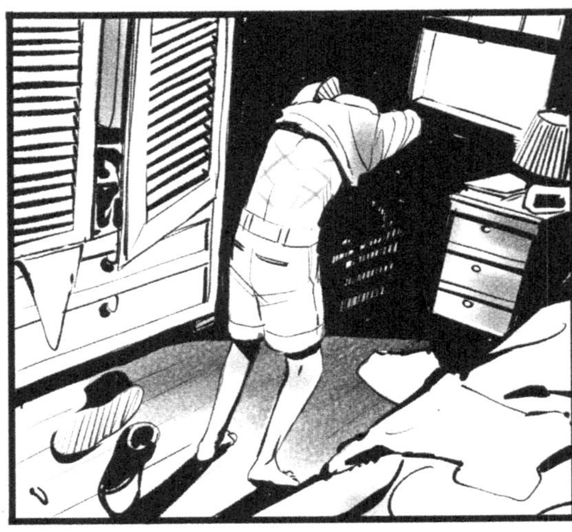

The sound of the running water filled the bathroom with a calming, white noise. I squinted, blurring my reflection in the mirror. That blur could be anyone. Whoever my imagination wanted him to be.

Usually, after one of my beatings, I would step into a cold shower and allow the cascading water to send me to someplace far away. It would wash over me as my mind willed it to wash away my very existence. I would step back out of the shower, with the welts already beginning to shrink some. Eventually, they would fade completely, leaving behind no evidence to be found except in my memory.

But this time was different. This time, I wasn't going to let anything *fade* away. I needed the evidence. No more hiding, no more concealing. This time, these bruises and welts would be worn like badges. I wanted them to be intact. I wanted them to be seen.

My perspective had shifted, so my actions needed to shift. Then, possibly, there was a chance that my life would shift as well. If there was any hope for change, I had to find my courage and reach out.

So this time, as I stepped into the shower, I didn't let the water actually touch me. I listened to the soothing sound of the droplets for a few more minutes, then stepped out and once again looked in the mirror. All the marks were still visible and my eyes had a steely new determination. My chin lifted a little bit higher, and my heart beat life back into my chest.

I got dressed to leave for church, but this time instead of the usual pants, I put on a pair of shorts. They stopped just above a large, purple bruise. A wave of anxiety rushed through me as I prayed she wouldn't notice. I was taking a huge risk in exposing her.

For all my nerves though, neither She nor anyone at church seemed to take notice of my bruises. If anyone really saw anything, they never said. After church, we headed to a birthday party at a local skating rink. Again, I did nothing to hide my injuries, and I would have been discouraged if not for a friend, Tyler, who *did* take notice, and talked to me about it. I found the courage to tell him what had happened, but I don't think he knew what to do with the information. Tyler left it alone and didn't ask me any more questions.

I was hopeful others saw the marks, that they noticed I wasn't okay anymore. I wasn't 'blending in' this time. I had to try because I truly needed help. I wanted them to see me for me, to know what I was going through. I needed someone to know that I was not okay.

When I got home that day, I had no regrets, but I did have an overwhelming fear sweep over me. What if I had made a terrible mistake? What if she had caught on and more beatings were going to follow? The wait was torture. I didn't know if anyone who mattered really noticed. Or cared. Were people that oblivious? Or was I invisible? Those were the wrong questions.

Despite my anxious thoughts, I made a plan. I was going to reach out to one more person. He was my last hope. And I knew he wouldn't let me suffer.

Would he?

# 13

# REACH OUT

didn't know if anyone else had noticed the marks I wanted people to see. It's possible someone saw and didn't feel comfortable saying anything. Some of the bruises could have been overlooked simply because I could have played roughly. That's not unusual. Many people are inexperienced at recognizing or dealing with signs of abuse. I will say, if you ever see marks on a person, trust your gut and say something like "What happened there?" Doesn't hurt to try and open a door to a conversation. Especially if they are a friend, reach out. Ask them if they're okay, or bring up your concerns privately to a teacher, counselor, or trustworthy adult. You might just be the hero they are searching for.

At this point in my journey, I was about to reach out to my father. I hoped he could be the support I needed. But a subtle enemy held me back. We all know its name and we've all felt its breath on the back of our necks. It's called 'Doubt,' and it's the ugly cousin of 'Fear.'

I had reached a point in my life where I needed to depend on others and go outside of my comfort zone. There's a heavy burden we often carry inside that makes us feel unworthy to take that first step. Whether it's going out of our way to ask a teacher for extra help, telling a parent how we feel, or even asking that cute classmate for their phone number, we feel that sense of doubt. It's a devious voice that keeps us from obtaining a goal or dealing with a difficult situation.

I was not okay with where my life was as a kid. And I didn't know if people would push me away once I shared my pain, but it's important for us to understand that we are never meant to get through the hardships of life alone. I escaped into sports in order to mask my pain. I discovered that being a part of something bigger than myself — and for you it may be a family, a team, or even the military — allowed me to focus on something better than my pain.

Kent Ferguson, a graduate from the University of Michigan and an Olympic diver from 1992 Barcelona Games, shared just how important a support system can be:

> I was not an athletic kid. I couldn't catch a ball, run a quarter of a mile without feeling like my lungs would burst, and I was always last to be picked on teams at school. I didn't like sports as a kid but my parents didn't give up on me. I was on the swimming team for a while, but swimming was too hard. I couldn't regulate my breathing and swim at the same time. It was discouraging.
>
> But the summer I told my parents that I wanted to quit the swimming team, my mom and

dad told me I had to do something active and not just sit around. For a kid who didn't like sports, how else was I supposed to have fun?

Well, I knew I really loved jumping on the trampoline, so my parents signed me up for lessons, an hour here and an hour there. Before long, I found myself on it hour after hour, day after day — and I even began competing. Everything about jumping was like nothing else I had tried prior in sports. There was an indescribable feeling when I jumped and soared into the air. The sensation of spinning, twisting, and controlling the movement of my body in the air was freeing.

When I was a competitive swimmer, I would find myself watching the diving competitions. It was hypnotizing. I had never tried diving before, and I wasn't sure it was something I could do. But then, just before entering my teen years, Eddie Cole, a part-time trampoline coach who owned an entertainment complex called Chapman's Fun World came into my life. He saw something in me at the trampoline gym that I didn't.

Volunteering his time, this world-caliber coach convinced me to try diving. Eddie, an NCAA champion diver and trampolinist himself, from the University of Michigan, paved a road for me that I never knew existed. It was a road that led me to the Olympics, where I learned that you don't have to win to be a winner.

What Kent and I both came to understand is that this world is full of people who are experts of their own experience; individuals who went through their own pains and struggles and successes. We all have a story, so it's important to know that even though you are the only one going through your story, it doesn't mean there aren't people who wouldn't understand. Trust me, there are people in your community who would definitely understand at least a portion of what you're going through. Had I not made the effort to get people to notice me, Doubt would have won and I would have lost.

Instead, I worked through the thoughts and feelings that were scrambling to hold me back, and I made the attempts to ask for help. Most importantly, I didn't give up, or come down hard on myself when the message wasn't received by others. What did happen, however, was that 'voice of Doubt' became quieter, allowing my courage to shine.

# OVERTIME REFLECTION

- Who has a positive impact on your life? Do they know how important they are to you?

- Who is a person you can trust that you can reach out to for support?

- What people in your life might benefit from your support?

# 14

# THE LEAP
# OF FAITH

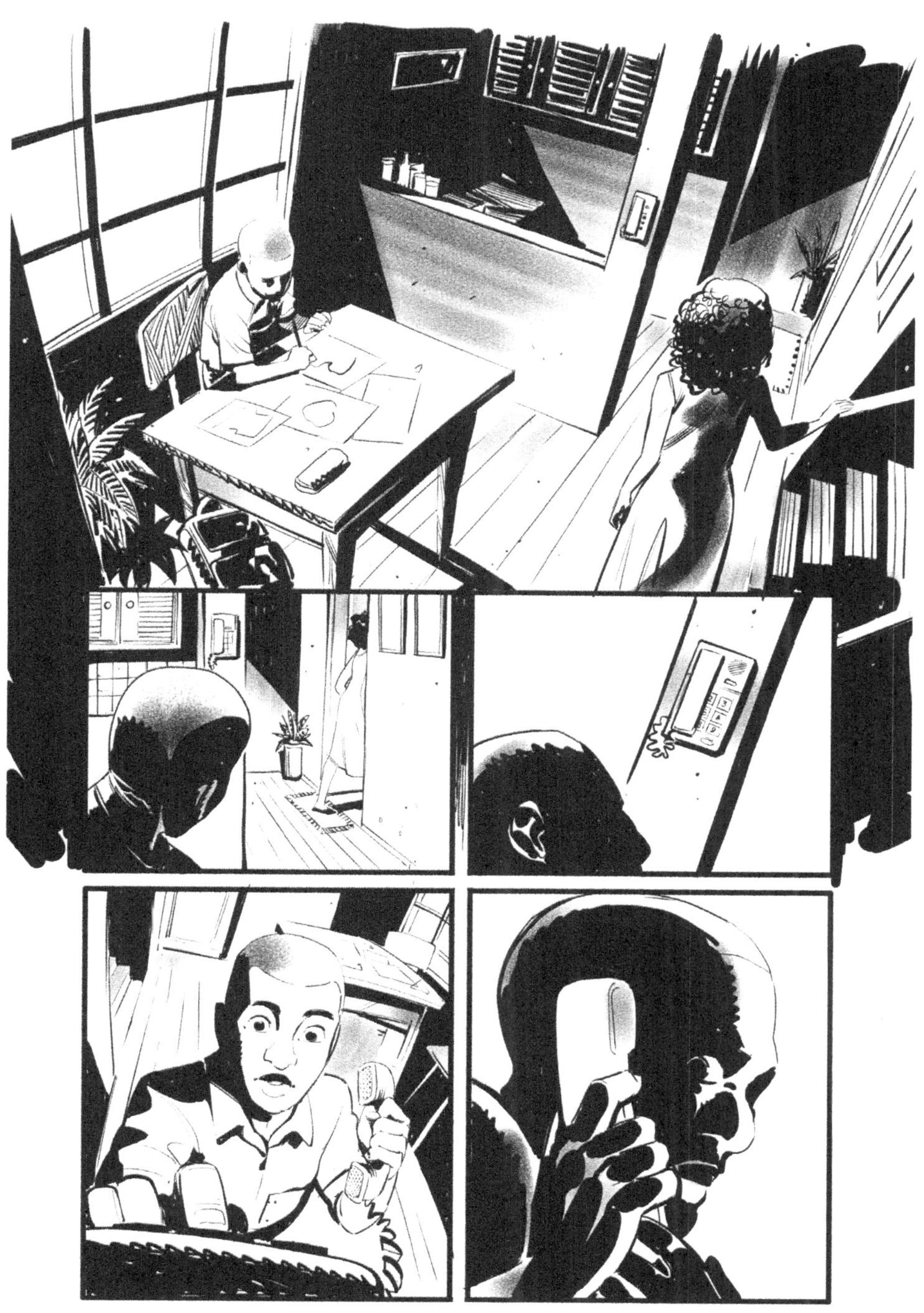

t was a Sunday night when I finally had a chance to call my dad. I had to wait until She was in the shower so the water would drown out any noise I might make. I couldn't let her hear me. Calling him was a 'no-no' here, so if I had an opening, then I needed to take it. I just stood there, staring at the phone in the dark, waiting for the faucet to run.

At the sound of the shower curtain swinging closed, I picked up the receiver and dialed. He had told me once, if I ever got a whuppin' bad enough to leave marks, I needed to tell him. After all this time, I was finally following through with his advice.

The phone rang …

And rang …

And rang …

He didn't pick up.

Slowly, silently, I put the phone back down and looked at it for another second or two. My heart beat a million beats-a-second. I anxiously picked up the phone again. My window of opportunity was closing fast, so I had to take the chance again. His number was one of only a few phone numbers I actually had memorized.

It rang over and over …

Still no answer. Each time it rang, I visualized him walking to his phone from the kitchen to pick up, but to my dismay he never did.

Before I hung up the phone, I heard his voice on the answering machine telling me to leave a message. Just the sound of his voice on the recording brought me back to a calmer state. I took a deep breath, but a rush of fear crashed back into me. Was she almost done?

I had to time out the message just right. I had to say the right words at the beep, and I had to do it fast. There wasn't much time left.

Oh, no! The water in the shower turned off.

*Beep*

The words spewed from my whispering lips as if in fast forward, "Hey, Dad, she gave me a whuppin' yesterday and I have marks on me."

I hung up the phone. Her door swung open. The light from the bathroom filled the hallway as she stood there drying her hair, staring at me.

"What are you doing?" She asked.

Staring back, trying to hide the fear on my face, I replied, "Nothing."

Before she could tell me where to go, I headed off to my room. The sheer disappointment of a failed opportunity hung on my mind, but that tiny voice deep inside said something else.

*"You did it. You got the message out. He'll hear it and you'll be safe."*

# 15

# HAVE FAITH IN YOURSELF

By this point in my life, I could have given up on fighting for myself. I could have left the ball in my dad's court and waited, sitting on my hands and hoping he would come to me. I could have beat myself up for even trying to put my neck out there. But all of those choices would have been wrong. I needed to take heart, to take control.

Because the more we allow fear, doubt, and anxiety to decide our actions, the harder it becomes to push through that discomfort. There comes a point in our life where we must face uncomfortable situations in order to grow. If you want to build muscle, you hit the gym and put your body through pain and discomfort. If you want to get your first job, you have to sit through an uncomfortable job interview where you 'sell your skills' and talk about yourself. If you want to play a sport well, you have to compete with people better than you.

Here are some more inspirational words from Kent Ferguson, the Olympic diver. He was one of the best of the best of the best, who competed against only top level athletes.

I didn't even classify myself as an actual "athlete" until after college — when I trained on the same team with four-time Olympic gold medalist Greg Louganis under six-time Olympic coach, Dr. Ron O'Brien. Ron truly taught us how to be athletes. He showed us what it took to think, train, eat, and focus like world-class competitors. I learned that while you don't have to win to be a winner, you do have to work hard to get where you want to go. That's when I really started to grow into the sport of diving. The passion started to increase as I mastered the sport, dive after dive after dive. I easily put in over 10,000 hours of time working on my skills.

But, I learned more from failing than winning. I didn't make the Olympic team straight out of college. In order to make the team, you have to be the 1st or 2nd best diver in the country. I was ranked #3 in the U.S. Olympic Trials. Four years later, after training 5 hours a day, 5 days a week, for 50 weeks, for four years, I tried out again, but still only took 3rd place, missing the Olympic team by mere points. So, thousands of hours and four years after that, I tried out a third time and made the team. After eight years of hard work and thousands of hours of training, I had finally done it.

I was 29 years old when I finally became an Olympic athlete, but it wasn't the outcome of the Olympics that mattered. It was the journey. I learned more about myself in those years of not being on the Olympic team than when I was on the team.

Look at Kent's example. He said he learned more from his failures than his wins. That means that every time he didn't quite succeed, he analyzed what didn't work, and tried to remove it from the next attempt. He knew he had to make changes and push harder than the previous dive. He had to make an effort to keep improving!

Lobsters shed their old shell to grow a new one because the space is too tight. Babies fall hundreds of times as they learn to walk. The body goes through pain in order to build muscle. The brain rewires itself in order to become sharper. A sword is forged through excessive heat and repetitive hits from a hammer.

Let's look at a tree or anything that starts as a seed. It begins in the dirt. It has to get dirty before it can grow. But the dirty part of its life is full of nutrients. It starts to grow, little by little. When the seed sprouts into a small tree, it faces harsh weather and all that nature can bring, yet it continues to grow. Then the storms come rolling in, so the roots deepen in order for it to withstand harsh winds. Then, it produces more seeds for the soil to nourish in order for more trees to grow. Trees know how to do life, and we can take so much from that.

When we see ourselves inside of this massive world, things may seem unwinnable. We may feel small and disposable. So let me just say that I felt that same way. But at some point I needed to have faith in myself and seek the potential inside of me. I had to start seeing myself as indispensable. I was not expendable. I wasn't a nobody. I needed to challenge who I was in order to be someone great. But even though life is dirty, we have to get through it in order to see what life has for us. A baby bird only knows the life within the egg, but when it comes out it discovers a whole new world of opportunity and adventure it never could have imagined.

As I began to make a stand for myself, I was finally seeing myself as important. I decided I had lived in a muddy swamp long enough. I pulled up anchor and began rowing towards wherever life would take me, away from the muck that was trying to hold me down. I see you just as valuable … just as priceless, and I encourage you to see that in yourself, too. Have faith in yourself even when times become too hard or when success seems like it's never going to come your way. Even if it seems like the sun isn't going to rise over the horizon, trust that it will.

Ask yourself, 'Why was I put on this world?' And then take that journey into self-discovery. Seek out knowledge through reading. Seek out wisdom through experience. Seek out success by failing. One breath at a time, one step at a time, one day at a time.

What we deal with inside of us — both good and bad — is contagious. We can spread love, fear, hate, joy, doubt, or excitement to the people around us. So take heart, be courageous, and have faith in yourself. Because when you do that, other people will have faith in you. And when that happens, people will start to have faith in themselves.

Be contagious.

## OVERTIME REFLECTION

- Do you believe in yourself, why or why not?

- What is something you know you're great at, and what is something you want to get better at?

- What is one way you hope to impact the world?

# 16

# MISSED MESSAGE

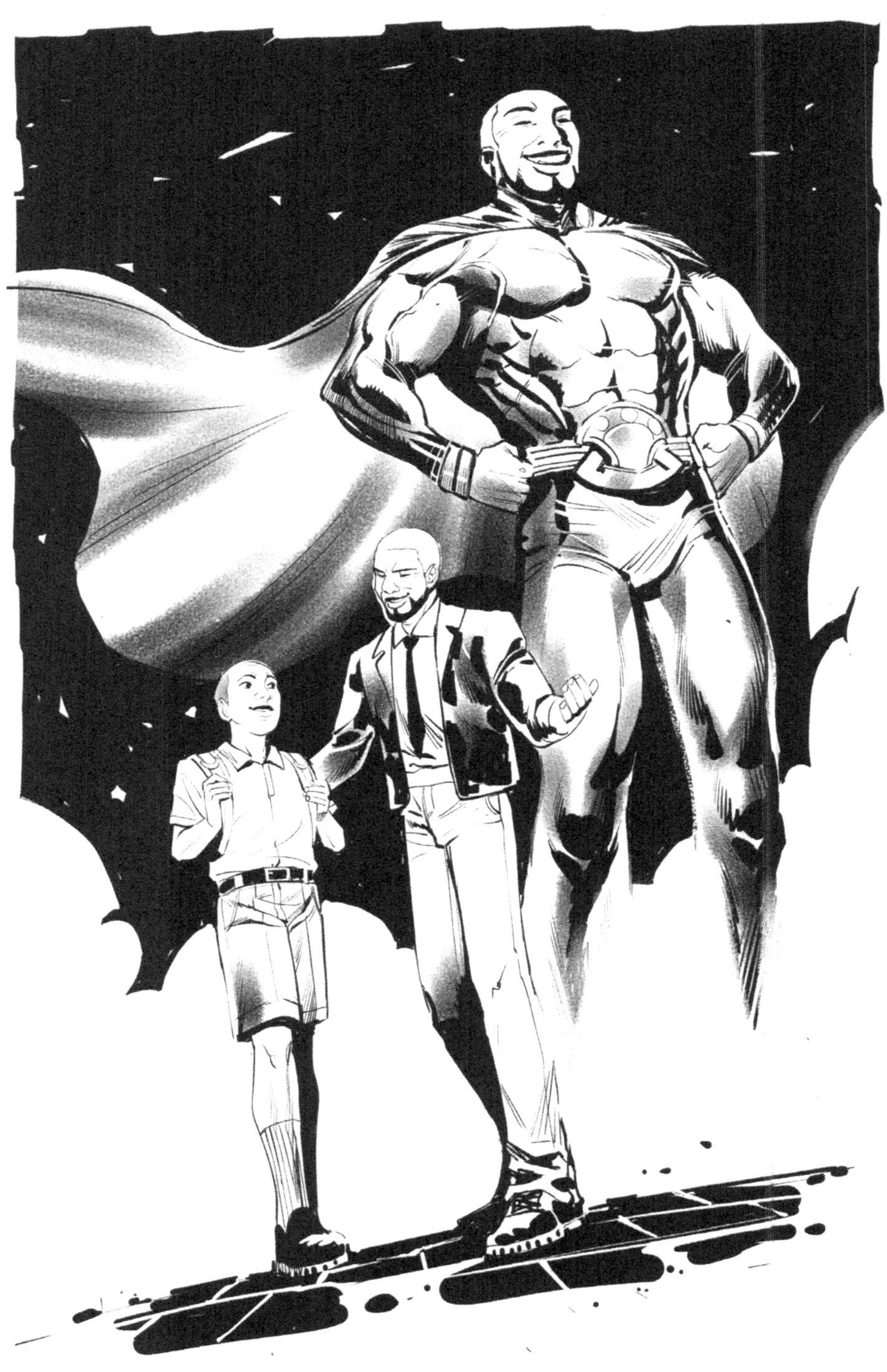

Talking to my father and seeing him were very important moments in my life. And whenever I was with him, he never wasted time. Our time together was more valuable to him than it was to me … … at first. But the more he pushed me to be better and not let life overcome me, the more I started to recognize the value myself.

When we were together, he was either helping me hone my skills, build my mind, strengthen my body, or fire up my spirit. I took great pleasure in counting down the days to when I'd get to see him again, keeping his words of encouragement locked inside my thoughts. I read the poems he gave me. I trusted the words he spoke. He was a strong foundation for me as a kid. It was vital for him to know what was going on with me. He only ever wanted me to be safe.

Our lives were complicated. I didn't get to see him as often as I needed to, and he knew this was a struggle for our relationship. A few years earlier, he had devised a plan to help me be able to communicate more effectively over the phone. This form of 'code talk' was a simple way for him to collect information about how my life was going under Her care. He knew there were few opportunities where we could talk in private, as all my calls to him were supervised by Her.

As I'm sure you've already gathered, my abuser was a person in my life who was supposed to be my caretaker. My father was aware that things were not ideal in that regard, but his hands were pretty tied. While he wasn't yet aware of the full extent of the situation I was dealing with, he had devised a secret code that allowed him to get more accurate, timely information from me.

"When are we going fishing?" meant that I hadn't eaten.

"Heading home from church..." told him when and where I was headed for the night. It also meant I hadn't done my homework yet, something he knew I couldn't reveal to Her.

These little phrases were simple messages he jotted down in his data log. He tracked all our phone calls, being sure to write down the dates, times, and duration of the calls. He noted everything important that I would say to him, how I sounded, and how long it took for him to call me back after he got a message.

When I had called and left a very direct, obvious voice message on his answering machine, he should have known something very serious had happened. I had never left a message like that before, because I was too terrified of the consequences if She found out. But this time was different because I had become important to myself. I wanted to live, and I wanted to live well.

I was devastated when I wasn't able to get a hold of him that Sunday. Not because I was giving up, but because the longer it took for him to get my message, the more my injuries would heal and fade. I needed him to see the bruises at their freshest.

I couldn't take pictures. No way. She would have found out. And I wasn't allowed to call him after my beatings because she was always still around. The bruises and fresh memories were always faded by the time we spoke.

I was just an eleven-year-old kid who didn't have access to my own phone. The only phones I could use were her cell phone and her house phone. She didn't let me be alone at church, except when I used the restroom. And I was always terrified to call Dad from the school phone. If someone overheard me say something like the voicemail I had left, she would have found out and everything would have been ruined. It was no easy task to tell your dad that you were being abused, with your abuser nearby.

My windows of opportunity were closing and I was losing heart. I feared she was going to win again.

# 17

# STAND UP FOR YOURSELF

can't reiterate enough how important you are. Sometimes — many times, in fact — things will appear gloomy and dark, but that doesn't mean settle within that gloom and wait for it to pass by. You fight your way through it, even if it's only you and the person in the mirror. When things go bad, when things get hard, when you get wronged, you stand and fight through. Your mind and heart are powerful tools, but so is your spirit! Unite all three parts and wield them in powerful and effective ways for your good. Don't just be motivated, be disciplined in what you want for yourself, in who you want to become.

A famous Greek poet named Pindar once said:

*Become who you are by learning who you are.*

Who are you as an individual? Do you love who you are or do you love who other people *think* you are? These are the right questions to ask. What is still missing in your life that is important enough to pursue?

In a world of 'cancel culture' and fear, where we often see people get shut down for making mistakes, or for just speaking truth, we have tricked ourselves into focusing on other people and their opinions. Too often it seems, some people feel more 'self-worth' when they are targeting the way others live, breathe, and believe. They feel better about themselves only if others are torn down. Somehow, for them, life has become a competition of who is right and wrong. We fall into the same trap when we compare ourselves with others, with people who set a standard that is very often not a good one. Why is that? We have tricked ourselves into believing the individual is not as valuable as the popular opinion or viewpoint. We've taken refuge under the wings of those who seem the most proud or confident. Sometimes, these people — though their presence is a comfort — distract us from really seeing who we are within ourselves. We become blinded to the one person who should matter to us the most. Take inspiration from people who are confident in their own identities, but do not try to *be* them, or please them. Just be you. C.S. Lewis had once said:

> A proud man is always looking down on things and people; and, of course, as long as you are looking down, you cannot see something that is above you.

If we are meant to stand up for ourselves, we can't do it with our heads down. Keep your head up, look towards the horizon, so you can better overcome the obstacles of the world around you. Take time to reflect when things become hard, and learn about who you are in the struggle.

Visualize this: We are like a strong ship on the ocean. When the storms of life come up, we seek a safe harbor where we can put down anchor. We try to stay grounded and ride it out. We can't control the weather, so we do whatever we can to just survive. But the storm grows bigger. The winds blow stronger and the lightning strikes closer, more frequently. The present troubles pile onto the past, and the waves of life begin crashing in on us from all sides. We must do something different, or we will sink! We have to weigh anchor and let the waves and wind pull us back out to sea! It's a terrible risk, but the storm would capsize us if we stay where we were.

For those who are still riding out that storm and just trying to stay afloat, don't stop. You cannot control the hurricane of your life, but you do have a say-so in what you do about it. I've heard motivational speakers say that life is 10% what happens to you, but 90% what you do about it. Keep seeking the change you need in your life, and before long you will see the light as you come out of the storm.

When I finally reached this point in the storm of my own life, I wasn't even a teenager yet, and I could barely see what life had to offer me. I wanted a better life, but wishing wasn't enough to make my desire come true. I had to take control and see the importance of being an overcomer; sitting in my past wasn't going to take me into my future. I had to take the step to call my father and leave the message for him. And when it didn't produce immediate results, I needed patience and resilience to not give up.

There is an epic story from the Bible where a young boy named David stood up against a giant named Goliath and won. One of the reasons he succeeded was because he understood what was inside him that no one else could see. Faith. Faith that he could overcome this mountainous man that so many other people feared. Practically everybody knows this story. Why? Because everyone can relate to the idea of being challenged by something too big and powerful to defeat. What is your Goliath? What towering obstacle are you facing that you have to get through, over, or around? Do you have the spirit to face those barriers and overcome them? You can't cancel or avoid all your struggles and hardships. Life comes with the good and the bad and the ugly.

For me, the hurricane was the abusive life I was stuck in. My *Goliath* was the fear I had to overcome. But once I began to understand the importance of placing value on my life, I also began to see that each day was an opportunity to grow, even when the battle was hard. I needed to be an overcomer.

There was no other option.

# OVERTIME REFLECTION

- What situations (if any) have knocked you down and kept you down?

- When have you done something well despite being afraid?

- What did those situations teach you about success? Did you grow from what you learned?

# 18

# DONT GIVE UP ON HOPE

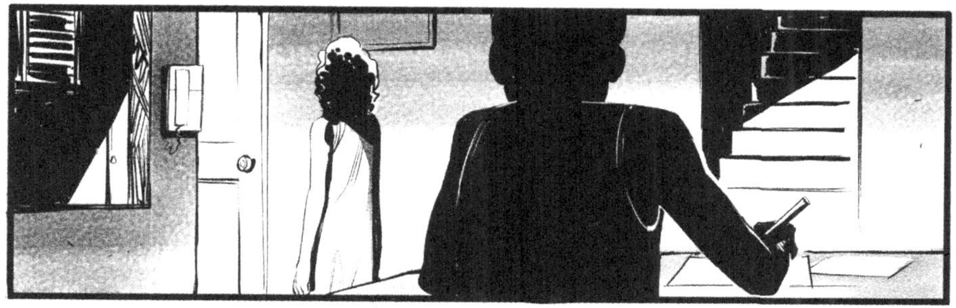
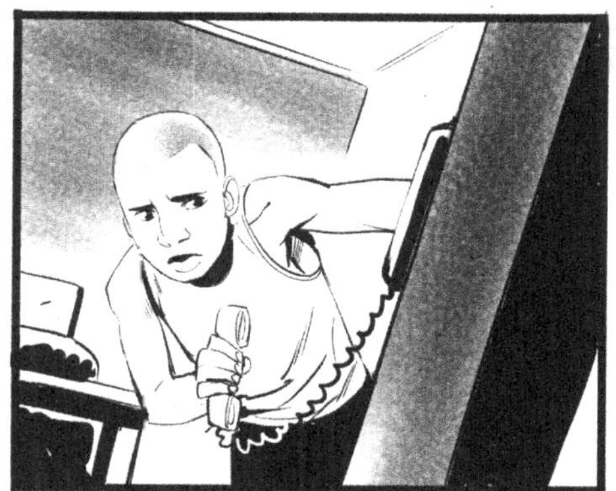
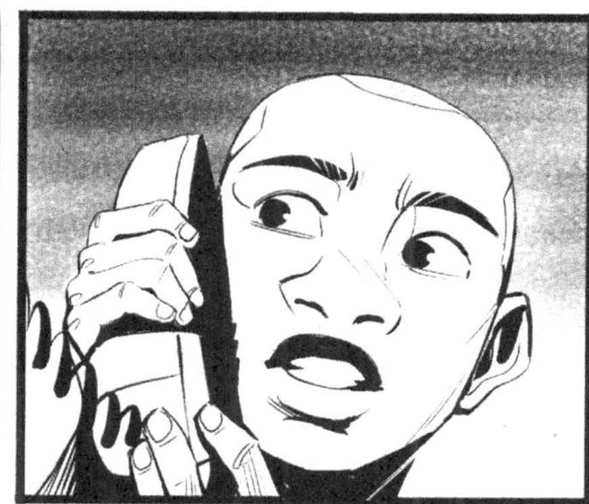
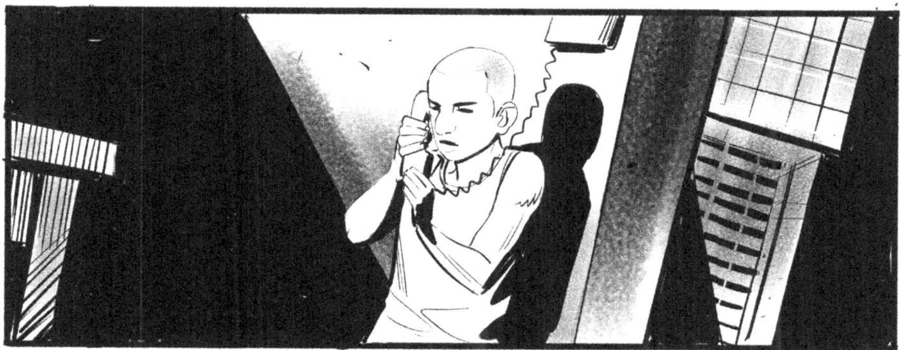
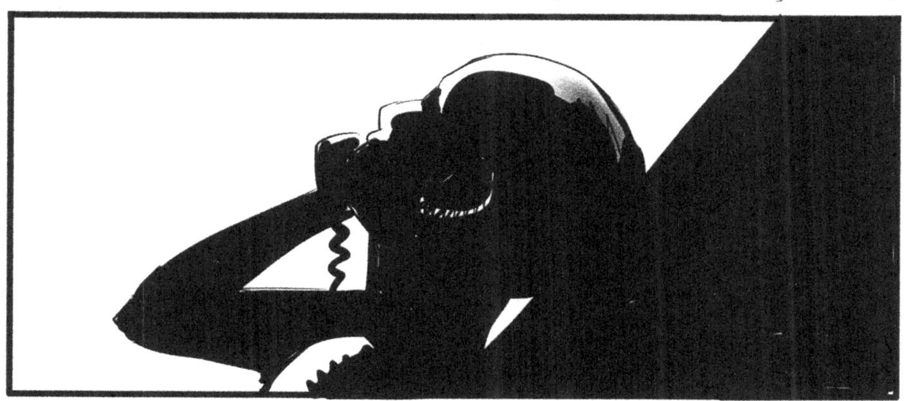

Two days later, a Tuesday, I was gifted with another chance to reach out for help. As the bruising and swelling continued to decrease, so was my window of opportunity. Once again, I had a chance while She showered. I picked up the phone and dialed Dad's number.

Once again, it rang. I held my breath, as if that might somehow help my chances.

It rang, and rang, and rang.

Then a click… "Hello?"

I let out my breath hastily, not wanting to waste any time. "Heeyy, Dad…"

"Hey, son," he replied, "How are you?"

I choked back hopeful tears. "I'm alright, Dad." I hesitated just for just a second before asking, "Did you hear the message I left you on Sunday?"

"No," he said. "I didn't."

*He didn't hear the message? How could he not hear that message?* I couldn't believe it.

"Did you need something?" he continued. "Need me to drop off some shoes?"

My heart was pounding. *Why hadn't he heard the message?* That question didn't matter now. I had no time to waste! Frantically, I took a breath and started, "I needed to tell you that—"

Suddenly the bedroom door swung open, and She emerged, dressed and ready for the day. The window of opportunity had slammed shut and I had failed to get the message to my dad for the second time.

I turned my back to her as a tear raced down my face. The disappointment slammed into my chest with gut wrenching force.I'd lost. I was still utterly alone.

Choking back sobs, I finished, "Okay, Dad. Well..." I didn't know what else to say, so I stuttered out, "I love you. I'll talk to you tomorrow." And hung up the phone.

I quickly wiped away all traces of tears, then turned to her and gave her the best reassuring smile I could muster.

But inside, I was broken. Time was running out.

........

The next day, I threw all caution to the wind. When she was in the shower I called my dad one more time. It was now or never. He *had* to help me. This wasn't how I wanted to live anymore. This wasn't the life I wanted for myself. I needed to trust someone.

The phone rang.

And rang.

Then *CLICK!*

"Hello?" he started.

I had to hurry this time. "Dad, did you hear my

message yet?!"

Slowly, he replied, "No, son, I haven't listened to it."

*Are you freakin' kidding me?!*

"Dad, she whupped me." I paused. The words were Truth themself, and a part of me finally felt comfort in being able to say it to him. "It was bad, Dad."

There was a long pause. He didn't say anything back.

I continued, "She left marks."

Another moment of silence between us on the phone. Time kept ticking and I was praying he was going to say something I desperately needed to hear.

"Son, I love you."

Nearly sobbing, I replied quietly, "I love you too, Dad."

A couple seconds later, he finally said, "I will be at your school at 9:00am tomorrow."

# 19

# FOLLOW THROUGH

When it comes to change and growth, it's extremely uncomfortable and difficult to do. That first step is usually extremely hard because it involves the conquering of fear. But just as difficult, can be the second step, which requires you to face doubt. But don't stop! Keep moving, keep progressing past these things, because *they* are not the whole journey.

One of the most vital parts to step one and two is following through. Committing to the change. Here's a small example. Let's say you're struggling with a class, or homework seems incomprehensible. You already know that if you don't seek change, nothing *will* change. Hiding the struggle or blaming the teacher won't create change. You have to be accountable for your actions.

So, Step One, reach out and ask for help. Don't hide it or keep it a secret, and don't blame the teacher. Let your teacher or a parent know you're struggling. Maybe it's because the work is over your head. Maybe you've been on your phone in class instead of listening. Maybe you missed a day of notes and needed to catch up. It doesn't matter the reason, as long as you hold yourself accountable and ask for help.

Step two, follow through. Be honest with them and yourself. Tell them your struggles and needs. Listen and learn. They are there to help you succeed. This is the job they signed up for, so show them that their extra effort to help you is worthwhile. Show them that you want to succeed. Stick with it and put in the work, and take responsibility where you may have willingly failed.

I can't tell you how common it is for people to fail to follow through. Many people don't even take that second step towards change. Their mindset is: "Well, I tried it and it didn't work." Or they expect someone else to fix all the problems *for* them. The doubt creeps in, causing setbacks. "Nothing works. I'm not good at this." And so many don't even want to make the first step. Not taking those steps is also a choice, but it is the wrong choice. Ultimately though, it's up to you to decide what you truly want from life. You cannot reach a destination just by wanting to.

Someone once said that the richest place on Earth is the graveyard. You'll find the most potential, the best inventions, and endless untapped creativity that was never spoken, created, or fulfilled. Why? Because so many people went their whole lives without taking the steps towards their purpose or dreams. Was it because they were full of fear or doubt? Were there circumstances in their lives that caused their dreams to fail? Do those questions really matter? No, they don't. What matters is asking the right question, about your own life. What can I do, to learn from the choices they didn't make?

What matters is *you* and what you do with your life *now*. Ask yourself: are you willing to take those first steps? The path will not be clear cut all the time. Many times, as long as you are moving forward, you'll come to a new "fork-in-the-road," a new choice that has to be made to decide your future. Those forks are not a place to plop down and wait idly. They are a time to continue working on ourselves internally and practice patience. There was a moment in my own life when I sustained a career-ending knee injury that took me out of the NFL. Up to that point, I had been working *towards* my football career, but now I had come to a fork... the path was changing and I had new choices to make. I had to be patient, work on myself, and find the next path that was meant for me. The end of my NFL career was not the end of my life, just the end of a chapter. The end of an era in your own life is not the end of the world.

As a young person, these decisions can appear colossal. And in a lot of ways they are! We know very little about what we're supposed to do, who we are, or where we're supposed to be. Our environment as a teenager is surrounded by different identities and distractions. It can seem unfair at times that so much of our future rides on the decisions of our youth, so sometimes we can be overwhelmed with what path to take. But just remember, you only need to take the first step. Work on yourself and understand who *you* are. Then the second step. Build your knowledge, skills, and support team. And then follow through after that. Don't give up, keep working, and take the path. You don't have to understand all the things coming, just understand that starting your feet on the right road will eventually take you where you need to go.

# OVERTIME REFLECTION

- What are your current distractions and bad habits?

- In what areas of your life is your discipline the weakest, and where is it the strongest?

- What daily routines can you start now to develop good habits?

# 20

## WHAT HOPE FEELS LIKE

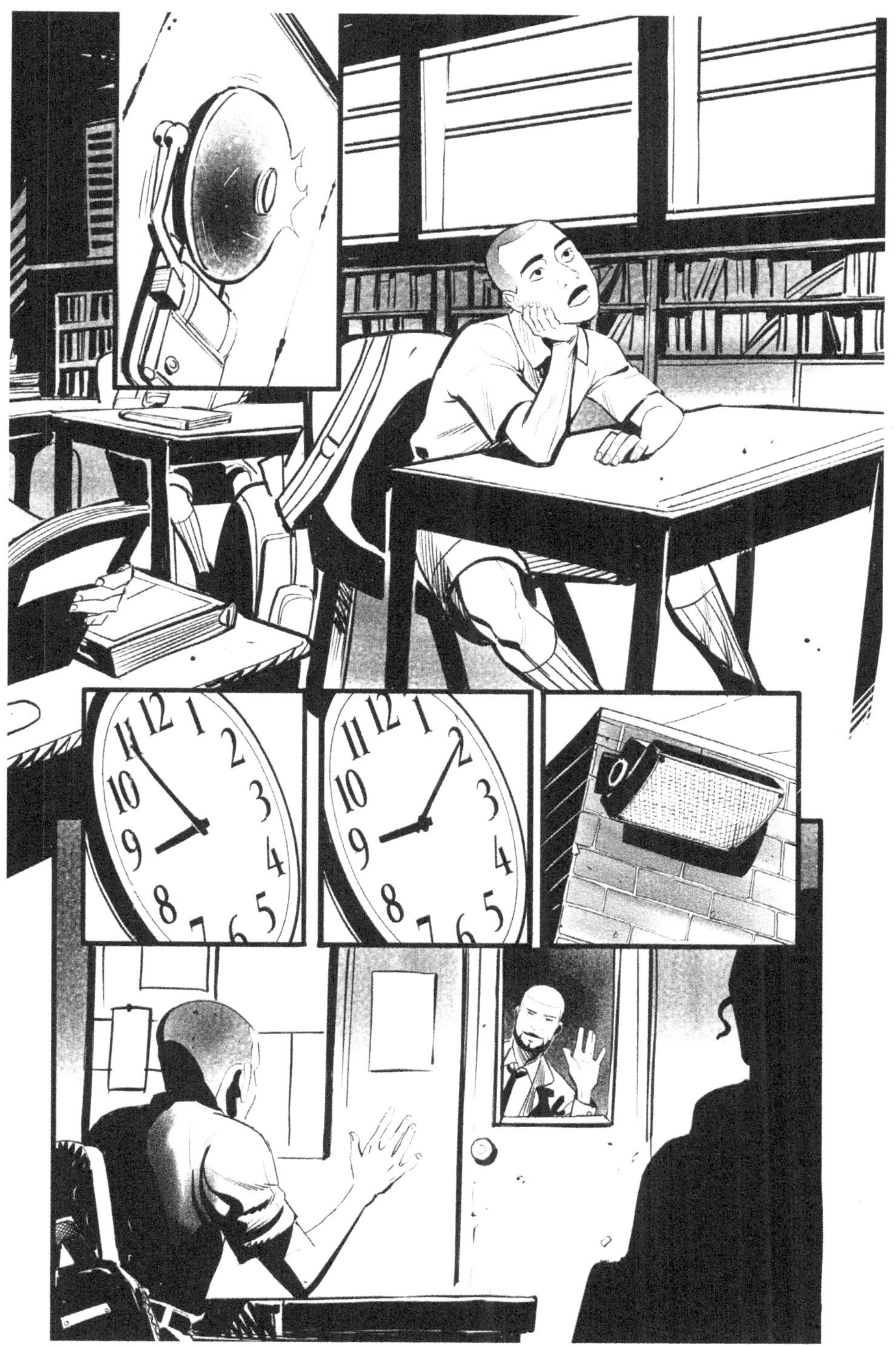

had never slept so well. Now that I had told my dad what had happened, I knew he was going to check the message. Speaking it out, using my voice to bring the abuse into the light, was very freeing. A weight had lifted. A large part of my mind opened up, and my body even felt lighter. Dad was going to come to the rescue in the morning, and things were looking brighter. Best of all, She had no idea. For once, I felt like I had the upper hand. I felt I had done right by myself, I was the master of my soul, the captain of my vessel. And for the first time I could say I felt safe. It was a breath of fresh air.

When school started, I was prepped and ready for him to arrive. Nothing was going to get me down, because there was a bright spot, a hero, my dad was on his way. I was a happy, nervous ball of energy. I wondered what was next. There were so many exciting questions in my head that went without answers. But the question that kept nibbling at the back of my joy was ... What if she found out?

As my 9:00 a.m. science class began, I couldn't hear a word my teacher was saying. My eyes were glued to the clock, my ears tuned to the speaker system. Any minute now I would be called out of class. If anyone around me noticed my anxious behaviors, I didn't care. I was poised and ready.

9:05 ticked by. Nothing.

9:10 — still nothing.

Maybe he was late. Or maybe he hit traffic. There was no way he would have forgotten about me, right? That wasn't his style. As doubt crept in I just focused on my bright spot. I kept up hope.

Then, at 9:15am, the squealing feedback of the intercom broke the silence. I held my breath, waiting for my name to be called.

"Asante … your dad is here."

I sucked in a huge breath, exhaled, and looked out the window to see his car in the parking lot. He had arrived!! Late as always, but here!

I couldn't help but note with relief that there was no sign of Her car. It meant that Dad hadn't said anything to her yet. The last time she had come to my school had been a really bad day.

It had happened a year ago. The night before a test, She had asked me if I had brought home my Math book to study. I hadn't. I had felt confident that I knew the material. She had then ominously stated that I had better *hope* for a perfect grade. I knew what she meant. This was a 'life test' and if I failed *her* test, she was bringing out the glue stick. The day after the Math test, she showed up at my school before the final bell had rung, went to my teacher's classroom, and asked about my grade. She didn't ask my teacher how I was doing in school or if I was a good student. She only asked about the grade on the test.

"Asante, did great. He got a 95%," the teacher exclaimed proudly.

But I saw the look on my abuser's face. I saw the rage behind those eyes. And I knew what was coming. When we got home that afternoon, because I hadn't gotten a 100% on that test, the glue stick came out and I got a beating.

But today, as I turned away from the window, there was my hero, framed in the doorway of my science class. I hadn't even bothered to unpack anything from my backpack when the class started, so I jumped out of my seat, picked up my bag, and ran to him. He hugged me tight.

I didn't care who saw. They didn't know what I was going through. I'm sure they knew something was up, my dad rarely showed up in the school. But it didn't matter. For now, he and I were in this together and I didn't feel so alone anymore.

The halls were empty. He walked me to the restroom and didn't say a word until we got there. He looked through the stalls to be sure we were alone before saying, "Let me see your bruises son."

I pulled up my shirt and showed him my back, then

rolled up my sleeves as he examined my arms. Without hesitating, I dropped my pants as he took in every mark on my legs. There was utter silence as I spun around, displaying all the marks that were still visible. This was the moment I had waited for, exposing the secrets underneath my long sleeves and fake smile.

I could tell that he was holding his breath. "Okay, pull your pants back up. I've seen enough." He was deep in thought. I couldn't tell if he was scared or angry or both.

With my eyes focused intently on his, I asked, "What happens now, Dad?"

Calmly and confidently, he replied, "Well, you go back to class. I'll take care of this."

I didn't know what he meant by that, but I knew I trusted him. I had to trust him. It was all I had to offer in support.

He walked me back down the hallway to class and gave me a quick goodbye. I snuck back into the room as curious faces peered in my direction. It felt strange to pretend like things were normal. But I did what he said. I went back to class and tried to act like a student who wasn't anxiously watching the clock again. Twenty minutes later the intercom squawked, "Asante, please come to the main office." Dad had been true to his word!

A few kids *ooh*ed and *ahh*ed at me, thinking I was

in trouble. A couple even snickered, but I didn't care. Not one bit. I'm sure my uncontrollable smile was confusing. They had no clue what was going on. Had I told them, it would have shut them up, but right now I needed to focus on the bright spots. I needed to listen to my dad and trust in what he was doing. With him here, my life was about to get better.

I entered the principal's office where a couple other kids sat waiting in chairs. The secretary kindly directed me past them and into a back office. I pushed open the door to find my father and the principal standing alongside her desk. All eyes were on me.

She smiled. "Come on in, Asante."

Two steps into the room, I turned and closed the door.

# 21

# HOW TO GROW

Everyone on the planet Earth will encounter influential life circumstances due to other people's effects on their lives. We cannot live without this happening at some point, both good and bad, and it's not something we can control. Whether these life-altering factors occurred from the time of pre-birth, childhood, or adulthood, we have all dealt with some sort of pain or struggle through no fault of our own. What I have learned in my own experience however, is that circumstance does not define us and pain is an integral part of life. It teaches us. It can either mold us into who we want to become, or into someone we weren't intended to be. It's our choice. We can't escape pain, it is a fact of life. But we can control our response.

I could have spent years pointing fingers and justifying and playing a victim. Who would blame me? But none of those options would have led to growth, resilience, discipline, or self-control. Those choices to use unhealthy pain to manage unhealthy pain, would have weakened and buried me. It wouldn't have helped me confront my circumstances. It would have kept me from growing.

Escaping your past and chasing down the future is so important when it comes to growth. We can only reach the future that we were destined to have by constantly growing and climbing. We all know that a plant cannot grow without first breaking out of its seed and then struggling up through the dirt and rocks towards the shining sun. If a plant wasn't willing to fight against the obstacles, it would never succeed in breaking out of the darkness and fulfilling its purpose. There has to be a point where we also acknowledge the obstacles in our way, but do not let them stop our growth towards our own purpose. If you choose to avoid the struggle, you'll stay in the darkness. It's a natural inclination we all have, to avoid pain, and unfortunately there are many unhealthy methods people use to try to feel only pleasure. It may sound strange, but avoiding ALL pain won't actually bring you life and purpose. The things worth fighting for will be hard.

Don't be distracted by things that don't help you grow. Distractions cause you to live life in contradiction to what your true purpose is, and can never bring you joy. I have never met a truly happy drug addict. Anyone fortunate enough to come out on the other side of addiction will tell you that at the time, it SEEMED like the drug solved the problem, but the minute the drug was gone, the problems remained. The only way they found peace and purpose was by facing the pain and growing past it.

You get one shot at life, so let's reduce the mess. Live your life *hard* by overcoming those barriers, but *wise*, by accepting your circumstance, and confronting your pain. I'm talking about school, home, relationships, work, sports, and within yourself. Because if you do, then life will actually be full of meaning.

As I stepped out into a new chapter in my life, I knew I had to be willing to overcome my hurt, so I could heal. It was going to be uncomfortable, so I had to take time to focus on myself in order to unleash the potential that was inside of me. I needed to shed layers, one at a time. I had to peel away my shell because I was going to grow.

The world will always be filled with darkness, wrath, tears, and pain, so don't expect it to go away. But William Ernest Henley said it best:

> Beyond this place of wrath and tears,
> looms but the horror of the shade,
> and yet the menace of the years,
> finds and shall find me unafraid.

Instead of succumbing to that darkness, we must change ourselves to change our lives. That means making conscious and deliberate decisions that push you towards your future.

I want you to know that it's not about what you look like or where you came from. It's not about how you were raised or if you have a disability or a special skill. It's not about how smart you are or how strong you are. Some have it harder than others. I'm not equalizing struggle, because none of us are the same, and no two people have the same exact future.

For example, look at a single-parent family with more than one child. Let's say there is no father in the picture and the mother struggles to keep food on the table. You'll notice each of the children will grow up to take different paths despite their similar circumstances of upbringing.

We can look at a family where both parents live in the home and have good jobs and a nice house. Again, you'll see that each child will have a different path than each other when they grow up into adulthood.

So what is the difference between individuals? Why do some succeed when others don't? That's the right question. Because of the choices they make for themselves.

Life is like a ladder we have to climb. While some people may have a nice, generic step-by-step plan laid out for them, that appears easy: get a job, go to college, get a better job, get married, have kids, retire, that may not be the ladder that's in front of you. There's nothing wrong with that generic plan, but what most people don't want to talk about are the barriers everyone's going to encounter on the climb.

Growth and discipline are not about taking a few steps up a ladder to do what everyone else is doing or what everyone else has done. Your ladder is yours alone, so just stay focused on your own climb. Don't let anyone else's doubts or expectations of you throw you off track. In fact, I challenge you to find the tallest ladder you can, with the most steps and the biggest future at the top and then just start climbing. And if you're scared of heights, then that is even more of a reason to find the biggest, baddest ladder. Why? Because you can never let doubt hinder your success. You are an overcomer that can and will climb to heights you never thought possible. You don't have to be ready for the top rung yet, just the one directly in front of you.

So pick a ladder and start climbing. Step one, step two, then follow through.

# OVERTIME REFLECTION

- What areas do you need to grow in the most?

- How can you turn your negative circumstance into a positive lesson?

- Are you truly willing to build resilience from your experiences?

# 22

# CHILD PROTECTIVE SERVICES

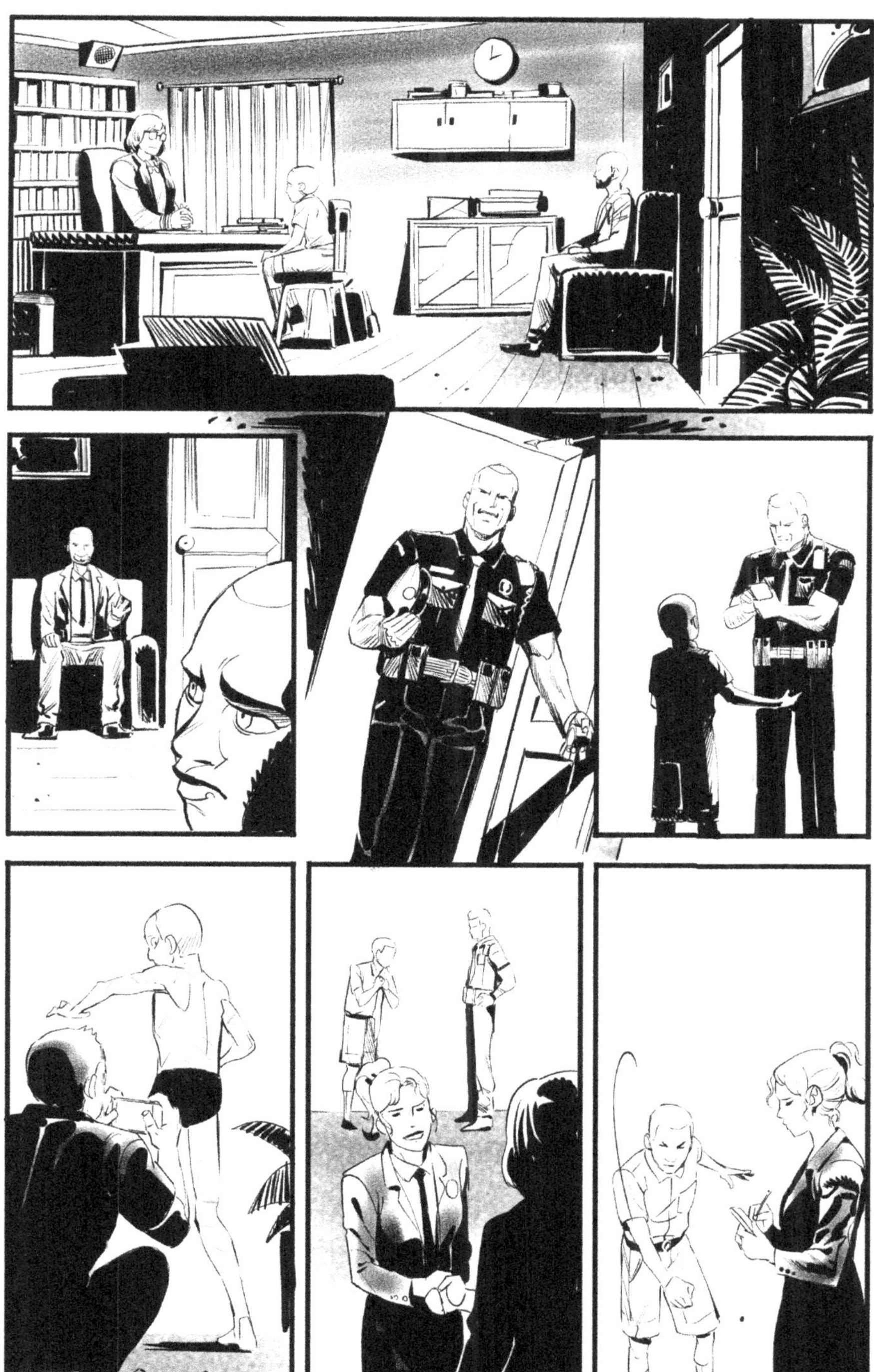

had been in this office before, but this time I felt hyper aware, like the room was brighter or more intense. As I sat down, the principal sat on her desk across from me. She had a good reputation at this school, but I didn't know her well. We didn't have much of a bond, so I was always hesitant to connect with her. I had never thought to trust her, but the expression on her face now showed genuine concern..

"Asante," she started, "your father told us everything. Because of what he said, I called Child Protective Services." She waited to see how I would react. "I also called the police station. An officer will be here shortly to take pictures and ask you a few questions, okay?"

I nodded, my eyes darting back and forth between her and my dad, who just sat there quietly. I can only imagine what must have been going through his own mind at that moment.

She asked, "Are you okay with that? I understand if it's a bit overwhelming right now."

"Sure." I looked again at my dad. His presence made me feel safer, calmer.

As if he knew what I was thinking, he added, "I have to go back to work now, but a friend of mine is going to pick you up."

That wasn't easy to hear, because I didn't want him to go, and I definitely didn't want to be with a stranger. I wanted to be with him. However, I trusted him enough to know he wasn't going to leave me in the hands of someone he didn't trust, so I took a deep breath and accepted his direction. With my Dad, the principal, and soon the police and Child Protective Services looking out for me now, I knew things were already beginning to look brighter.

Rather than spend all day waiting in the office for the various people to arrive, I had to return to my classes. So, throughout the school day, the overhead speaker kept blasting, "Asante to the office" or "Asante, would you come to the office, please?"

Kids were curious, and some even asked me what was going on, but I just smiled and went about my day, doing as my father and principal instructed. What would I have told them? And how would I have said it? Right now, I didn't want to risk anything or be stupid. I just did what I was told - whether I knew all the answers or not.

When the police arrived, they spent a lot of time questioning me. I told them my story over and over again, shining light on everything that happened behind closed doors. They didn't want to miss a single detail. The more I talked about it, the easier it was to say aloud. I was freeing myself from a weight I had carried for so long.

I showed them my bruises and marks more than once as they photographed each and every one. I didn't even hesitate to pull down my pants.

Sometimes, flashes of the abuse would hit my thoughts, but as I talked about it more and more, my mind became clearer. It was like letting go of a heavy burden. I knew what was at stake and I needed them to see what was done to me. I trusted these strangers with my vulnerability, because my father trusted them.

Child Protective Services also thoroughly questioned me. Their questions were very direct as they went through my story with me. Again, I didn't leave out a single detail. And just like with the police officer, not a single mark or bruise was overlooked when the human service worker took pictures.

By the end of the day, I was completely exhausted from all the talking and processing. My adrenaline and anxiety had been at a max throughout most of the school day. When the final bell rang, I had given them everything about my life story. Now I simply had to wait and see what would happen next.

As always, the bus headed to drop me off at my old elementary school. I ignored all the energetic kids around me as my mind began to fixate on one worried thought. My abuser was usually the one who picked me up from school.

She had no idea what had happened at the school (I hoped) but I didn't know what to expect when I exited the bus.

*What if she showed up to pick me up? Or was she already waiting for me?*

# 23

## SOMETIMES THERE ARE DETOURS

**I**f you've ever played online video games, you probably noticed how rarely each match goes your way. You enter a virtual world with other people who have a variety of skill sets. From the time the game starts until it ends, everyone has choices to make. These choices lead to their actions. Their actions lead to different outcomes. No two players are able to perform the exact same way.

The same goes for sports. As an athlete, we know that practice sharpens our skills. And in each game, we do our best to make the right choices each second, inning, round, and quarter. Yet, there are times things won't play out the way we hoped they would. A missed goal, a dropped pass, an error, or missed shot. One single mistake could cost us the game. And *that's* the important thing about life.

Life is the same way, it's never consistent. Wins and losses will vary. Sometimes we won't see the loss coming — a failed grade, a breakup, a divorce, a death, or a career-ending injury. These things happen. It's life. Life is unpredictable and hard and overwhelming at times.

We can't possibly know how every day ahead of us will go. Perfection doesn't exist, no matter how hard we try. Yet, every second of every day we have choices to make. These choices are what lead us in one direction or another.

Sometimes we intend to do good, but it ends badly for us. Sometimes, we're in the wrong place at the wrong time. And sometimes, life just decides to throw us options we are unprepared for.

These decisions we make day-in and day-out can become a pattern — habits, good or bad. These habits take us through different paths with different circumstances and different outcomes. Bad habits can destroy our reputation, our career, our relationships, or our will to live. Some lead us to jail, abusive partners, addictions, or worse. And sometimes, it's not just one choice that hurts us, but a conglomeration of many choices. There are times we spiral out of control, and we don't even realize it until months or even years later.

So these moments, where life throws us a curveball, veering us in a direction we never wanted to go. How do we respond?

That's the right question. Up until the point that Child Protective Services (CPS) came into my life, I had been making some choices in my own life that were detrimental to myself. No, I was not responsible for the abuse happening to me, but I was choosing to keep silent about it. Had I *not* made the choice I did to step out, afraid but courageous, and tell my dad the truth, there's no knowing where my path would have taken me. Allowing CPS to make a decision for me, was the best choice I could have made. I experienced trauma, I found a bright spot, I utilized my voice, and I trusted their decision on what would happen next.

This sudden shift not only impacted my life, but it impacted all the things going on inside my body. All those old habitual thoughts and feelings still existed, and they carried a residue of fear with them, because change is hard. I didn't have any of the answers to "What's next?" or "What if..." or "Now what?" I didn't even know if things were going back to normal. All I knew was that there were other people in my corner, working to help me.

I want to acknowledge that there are sometimes situations that occur in other people's lives that aren't as quickly resolved as my own experience. Sometimes a bad situation — one you can't control — can cause a more drawn out life battle — the death of a loved one, sexual assault, a life-altering injury, someone taking advantage of you, or simply a phone call with terrible news coming from the other end. Sometimes these events can completely destroy our philosophy — the way we see ourselves and the way we see the world around us. We start to blame ourselves for why this is happening, or we say that this is something we deserve. These negative ways of thinking are dangerous and will cripple your progress if they become a habit. So how do we adjust? How do we move through it?

One way we can prevent a bad turn of events from worsening — or becoming too overwhelming to bear — is by taking action. We need to plant new seeds. We have to cope and process the life-altering event. Avoidance never makes it go away, it only draws out the pain longer. If this is you, reach out to the school counselor or talk to a teacher after school — a neutral party will be able to find resources or be a safe ear to talk to. If you are connected to a local church, reach out to a spiritual leader there. Find that person that can offer you the healthy emotional, mental, and physical support you need. We need to get our mind right, to remember who we are. Journal and process and be mindful of your current situation. Ground yourself in the moment. Maybe we need to heal — mentally, physically, or spiritually. Whatever it is, do it on purpose. And be patient. For some of us, it will take time to bounce back.

In August of 2020, during the COVID-19 pandemic, a derecho swept across Nebraska, Iowa, Wisconsin, Illinois, and Indiana, causing devastating damage. Unlike a rotating tornado or hurricane, a derecho's winds blow in a straight line, accompanied by thunderstorms, over great distances. Usually, derecho winds blow 55 to 70 mph.  During this particular derecho, winds got up over 120 miles per hour in some places – the same speed as a category three hurricane! Hundreds of thousands of people lost electricity, some of them for several weeks! It did eleven billion dollars' worth of damage. Trees were torn from the ground, homes destroyed, jobs lost, and lives ruined. It was devastating to see.

But something that resonated with me was how quickly the majority of Iowans responded to the life-altering event with positive action. There were stories of neighbors meeting neighbors for the first time, helping each other out of the destruction. Chainsaws ran from dawn until dusk for weeks, cutting up fallen trees so roads could be cleared, electricity restored, repairs begun. People supported their local businesses and local businesses supported the people. People made gas-runs to neighboring cities just to keep the work going. When the stores ran out of lumber, people with trailers delivered it from as far away as Kansas City and Omaha. Online resources for help and communication sprang up practically overnight. It was incredible.

Iowans didn't sit idly by. They didn't wait for others to pull them out. They didn't allow this to cripple them. And while they certainly asked for and were overwhelmingly grateful to accept outside help, they didn't wait around for anything to be done for them. They maintained their philosophy of who they were as a state. No matter the disaster, they weren't going to stay down for long. Many people in Cedar Rapids were hard hit by the derecho while still trying to recover from the flood of 2008, but did they give up? No! As hard as life became for them, they endured.

By making conscious choices every day to change and process and overcome the unexpected, we too will be able to adapt. We'll be able to shift some things to our advantage. Over time, we can form newer and better habits. As these habits continue, we can grow. We can't allow ourselves to become content or to just maintain. From struggle, there is growth.

It wasn't easy for me, and it's probably not easy for you — whoever you are, going through whatever you're dealing with. Maybe there are stories you've seen, heard, or read about where people bounced back from insurmountable struggles and failures. And maybe it's something you don't believe you're capable of performing. Well, I'm here to say it's possible. I'm living proof. So I want you to look deep down inside yourself and to see that strength you have. It's there, waving its hand at you. Make it happen, start planting your seeds, tending to them, and growing through the struggle.

Just remember, when life delivers a sudden sourness, don't let the taste settle. It's not something to savor. Spit it out and find something better to chew on. You deserve better, so fill your belly with something nourishing, good, and healthy for you. There is strength inside of you. Find it.

# OVERTIME REFLECTION

- Has life ever put you in situations that are out of your control?

- How does change make you feel?

- What is something you want to change in your life?

# 24

# HIGH ALERT

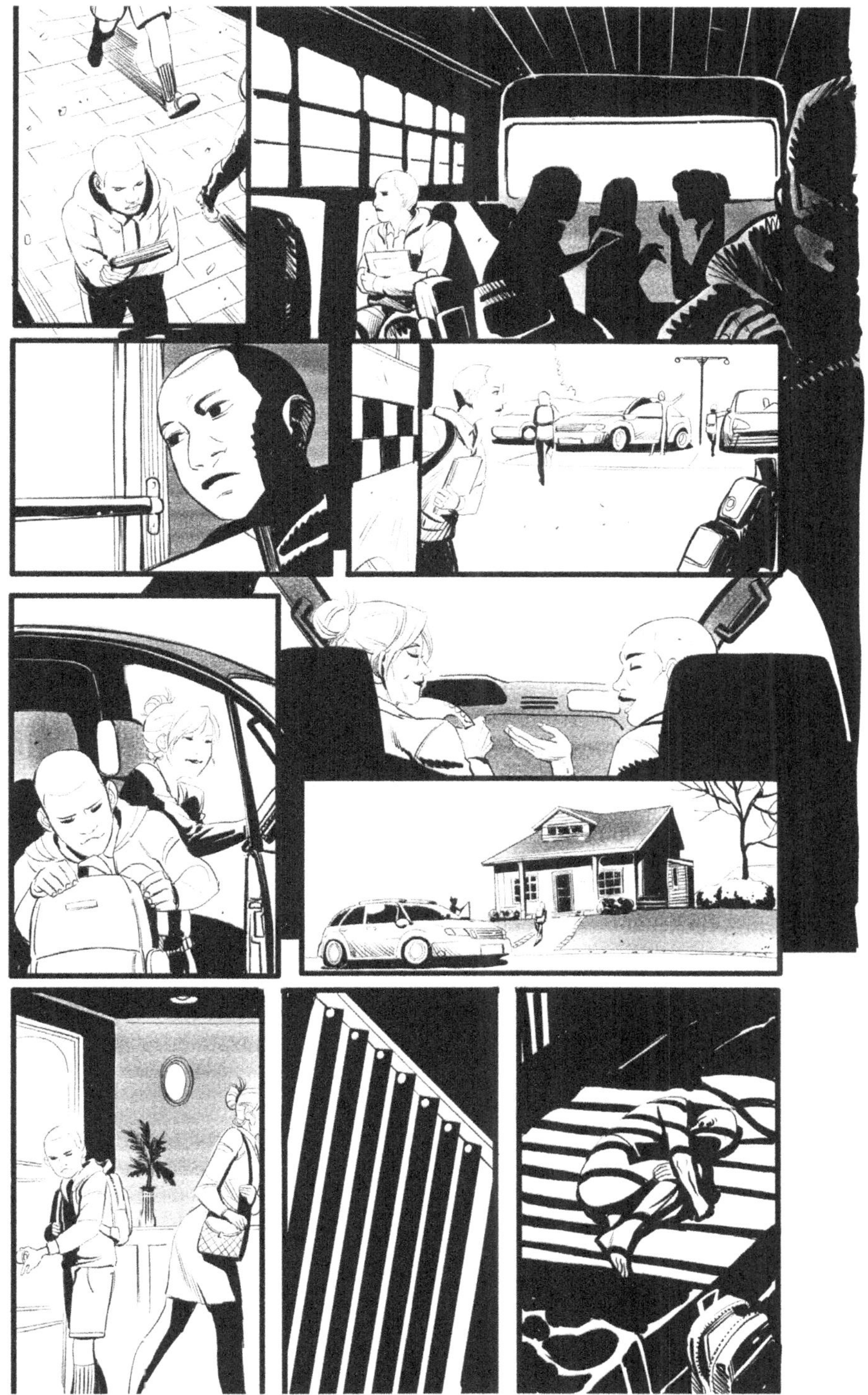

Still oblivious to the other kids around me, I anxiously scanned the parking lot for my abuser's vehicle as the bus came to a full stop. My beating heart kept me grounded to my seat as the other students walked past me like I was invisible. As if on auto pilot, I somehow exited the bus myself. The kids running to their parents' vehicles felt like an alternate world overlapping my own. I barely noticed them as my mind was fixated on one thought, and one thought alone.

Then, I saw her. No, not my abuser, a teacher, Mrs. Rice, from my old elementary school and a friend of my father's. She was waving to me from her car, telling me she was supposed to take me to my dad's house. My heart leapt into my throat and I hurriedly jumped into her vehicle, cradling my bag, and then the dam burst and I began to spill my guts. I mean spilled them. You would have thought I had revealed enough already today, but nope … my story was still begging to be told. The words ran off my tongue like an assembly line.

I told the poor woman everything. I didn't know if she already knew my story, but there was no escape for her, stuck in this vehicle with me until I got to my dad's house. I rattled off my entire life right up to the point where the police took pictures of my naked body. She listened to every word and by the look on her face, I'm pretty sure I freaked her out. She had no idea what she had gotten herself into.

Because of all the practice talking with my father, the principal, Child Protective Services, and the police, I had mastered my story. It was getting easier to tell, but at the same time my body was still riddled with anxiety and adrenaline. On the outside, I was tense and fidgety. On the inside, I was absolutely terrified that my abuser was going to come after me. I didn't put it past her to come to my father's house.

"She might have a swat team come through the windows to get me, you have to be prepared," I added as I finished up my story.

Mrs. Rice was speechless, but I had no idea what lengths my abuser would take to get me back. I believed the whole 'swat team' thing, too. I envisioned a huge black truck stopping in front of my dad's house. The back doors swung open and a team of armored enforcers spewed out with guns at the ready. My heart beat like a wild drum as I thought about them busting in the front door and taking me back as I kicked and screamed.

"We need to be on high alert," I continued. "Ready for anything."

I couldn't slow down. There was no staying calm.

The anxiety and adrenaline put my worries and fears on overload. I'm sure she thought I was hyped up on energy drinks, or just out of my mind, but I couldn't sit still or focus on one single thing. My thoughts, chemicals, and body were completely dysregulated, which was why going to my father's place was going to be so good. I needed a place to be safe and to process everything that had happened to me so far.

When we arrived at my dad's, I sprinted ahead of her for the front door. Opening the door, I threw my bag, then turned, and locked the door the second Mrs. Rice was inside. Then I ran and checked all the windows and closed the curtains. Regardless of what my old teacher thought. I had to make this place feel like a fortress against encroaching enemies. Subconsciously, this was what I needed to feel safer. And it did. Though it was probably irrational, in my head it was a necessity. Mrs. Rice left me to myself to settle in while we waited for my dad to get off work.

Waiting felt like an eternity. I didn't use the restroom or get anything to eat. I didn't want anyone to know I was here. I didn't want Her to know I was here. And I was petrified. The fear of my abuser busting in the door and taking me sat heavy at the front of my mind. I was anxious inside and out. Who knew what would happen next. Each time a car drove by, a door closed, a horn blared, I tensed up more and more.

The ticking clock and my beating heart made every second seem endless. I had never wished for time to fast forward as badly as I did right then. I wanted my dad here. He would make it all okay. I wanted to feel okay.

At long last, Dad came through the door from work. My hero had made it. The room instantly became more secure, feeling nearly impenetrable. He was like the 'David' to the 'Goliath' of my fear. As Mrs. Rice quietly left, I was able to get up from my spot and move around with a little less anxiety. I followed him around like a shadow for a bit until I could feel myself becoming more regulated.

He moved about the house like there was nothing wrong; completely calm and collected. I think he knew the level of stress I was under, and his calm demeanor soothed me visibly. I began to talk to him.

"So, do I live here with you now, Dad?"

He looked at me and then came close to where I stood. "Well, Son, would you like to?" he inquired.

That question was a breath of fresh air. Knowing this was possible, I could breathe freely again. A smile stretched from one side of my face to the other. There was nothing that I wanted more in the world than to live with him.

"Yeah, Dad, I would like that a lot."

I couldn't contain my happiness. Or was this emotion

called joy? It didn't matter. I was in the clouds now. For once, I felt safer than safe.

"I'd like that a lot too, Son."

That night, he took me out for pizza. It was the first time that we had eaten at this particular restaurant, Round Table Pizza, and it was the best pizza I had ever or will ever eat in my life. Freedom never tasted so good. Somehow, when things are looking up, everything seems better in its own way.

I could only pray that this was permanent.

# 25

# DON'T CARRY ANXIETY

The weight of anxiety is a heavy burden, and shedding that weight is one of the toughest things to do. It's not something you can just 'let go' because that's not really how it works. Telling someone to stay calm is rarely an effective way to help with anxiety, no matter how many cool shirts and memes you see. In my decades of life, never once have I seen someone overwhelmed and anxious actually calm down instantly after being told, "You should just calm down."

Anxiety can strike almost at any time, like when raising your hand in class, or talking to someone you're attracted to, or just standing next to a stranger on the subway. These may sound like small things to some people, but for those living with 'survivor brain,' they are huge challenges! Anxiety can be quite harmful if not put in check.

There are times when anxiety can be attached to hard things also, like going to school every day and hoping no one knows you're homeless, or going to the home where your abuser lives, or telling a loved one or counselor that you are not doing okay mentally or emotionally.

It's okay to not be okay.

Let me say that again: it's okay to not be okay.  It's

okay if you are unhappy and angry that your hair has fallen out of the style you spent so long putting it in. It's okay if you're disappointed you didn't score well on the last test. It's okay if you're scared of being bullied because you're new, smart, overweight, skinny, have an accent, or whatever else makes you different. It's okay if you're upset because someone said they didn't want to be your friend. It's okay if you're just frustrated because life is hard and it feels like you're the unluckiest person in the world.

However, it's *not* okay to keep it to yourself. You have value and you have a voice, so stand up for yourself and protect yourself because you are a treasure to this world. You are beautifully and wonderfully made. You have something to offer this world, so let's get to a point where you can share your gifts with the world confidently.

When we look at anxiety as a whole, we know there are different degrees of it, and people will experience it in a variety of different ways. What many of us don't do is bring those feelings to the forefront of our daily routine where we can cope, regulate, and process through it. We sometimes just wait for time to get us to that next moment in the day so we can think a little bit clearer. Let's be real here, anxiety has even become a type of "socially acceptable" challenge that sometimes we even use to fuel us through our day — on social media, in simple conversations, or through relationships. But that's not a healthy lifestyle plan. Over time, anxiety will eat away at the gifts you have to offer this world. It will attempt to cripple you, so you can't affect the world for good. It is not your friend, even if it's familiar. There is much, much more for you beyond it. Finding ways to minimize its effects on your mind and body will be well worth the effort.

Over my years of dealing with my trauma, I needed to take time in my daily routine to recognize how to overcome those anxieties that had scarred my spirit. There were moments where I could handle it, but then there were days it would strike quick and fast like a lunging cobra. And if I wasn't ready for it, I got bit.

There are many ways to help with anxiety, different coping tools to incorporate into your daily routine. Breathing techniques are my go-to, all the time. There are so many benefits of intentional breath-work: calmness, focus, clarity, and even patience. What are some activities you can do that will integrate breathing simulations? For example, guided meditation and exercise. Both involve conscious breathing and body awareness.

There are simple techniques of inhaling slowly for four seconds and exhaling for eight seconds in order to regulate the heart rate and blood pressure. Yoga embraces thought-processing skills, body awareness, and breathing techniques that people throw into their daily routines.

How else can you practice different breathing styles? Going for a run or a walk, or even hitting the gym. If you don't have access to these things, then ask the school teachers if they can facilitate after-school yoga classes or gym workouts. Ask a coach if you can utilize the school weight room. Again, there are numerous ways of doing simple, independent breathing techniques by sitting in your chair or on your bed, or when you're being active. Pick one, and stick with it. See what style fits your personality.

And there are, of course, other ways to battle your anxiety — focusing on your self-care. Journaling is a great way to consciously process your thoughts and feelings. Start a good sleep routine. Find ways to improve your diet. Decrease your use of electronic devices (especially at bedtime) and replace that time with books; expand your literary world. Build your self-confidence daily, set goals, and work on yourself when no one else is looking. You do you.

If you find yourself thinking this all sounds like work, you're right. It is! As I've said before, anything worth doing requires effort. It also requires belief in yourself and your worth. You may not be fully convinced at the start that it will work, or that you deserve to feel better, but the fact is you *do,* and it *will.* We only grow with effort, we only change by making new choices, and the more we work at anything, the stronger we become. The stronger we become, the easier it is to do more things. Start small and work your way up. Any true effort will make a difference!

The more you take time to recognize and address your anxiety, the more you'll put focus and confidence into overcoming it. Invest in yourself. Be the better version of yourself. Love who you are. Discover who you want to be. Identities are everywhere, but there is only one that fits you, and you'll find it along the path to doing what you were meant to be doing.

Why is self-confidence such a big deal? Well, because if we don't have self-confidence, what else is left to fill its place? Depression. Anxiety. Fear. A sense of meaninglessness. The list goes on. But something else is just as important as self-confidence; self-worth. Eliminate the two, and life can be hard to balance and full of emotional obstacles. But, if you develop self-confidence and self-worth, it's like putting armor on a confident warrior. It's both interior and exterior strength and protection.

And the more you feel confidence grow, the more you'll act like it. The more you act like it, the more that confidence becomes a habit. Habits like this can build into something even more powerful, resilience. As things come at you, you'll have the emotional skills to deflect and protect yourself against the offense. You'll be able to bounce back quickly and be back in the game without missing any play.

Chip away at it every single day. Life isn't going to serve you success on a silver platter. You need to work for it, and it'll be tough, but in the end it will be worth it.

Anxiety tries to make us feel small in this world and it takes up too much space within our mind, our body, and our spirit, so it's time for you to limit its space inside of you. As you keep at it, you'll start to have more room in your life to think about your dreams, desires, hopes, and aspirations. They won't seem as impossible anymore.

And someday you are going to become that *someone* you have always dreamed of becoming. Have courage and don't be disheartened. Hope that you will be that somebody you were always meant to be.

I believe in you. Don't give up.

# OVERTIME REFLECTION

- How do you behave when you're overwhelmed?

- What is the root of your anxiety?

- What methods or tools can you use to build your sense of self-worth?

# 26

# FACING MY FEAR

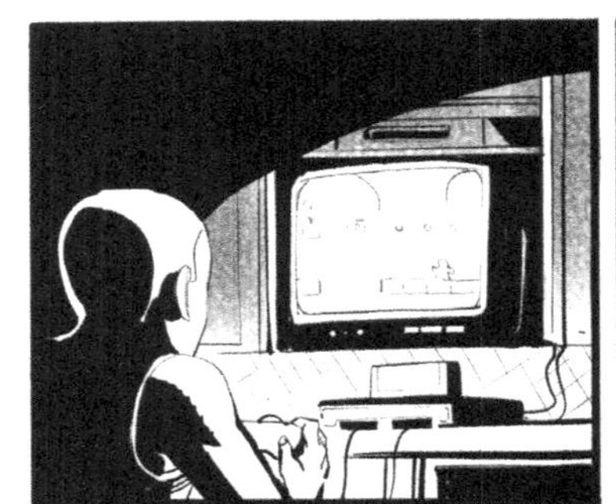
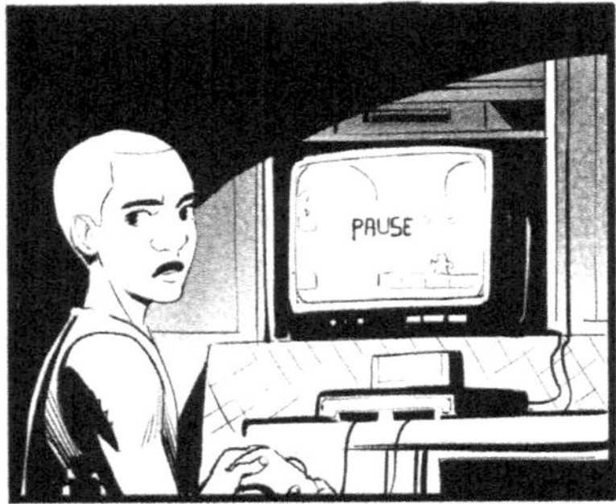
PAUSE
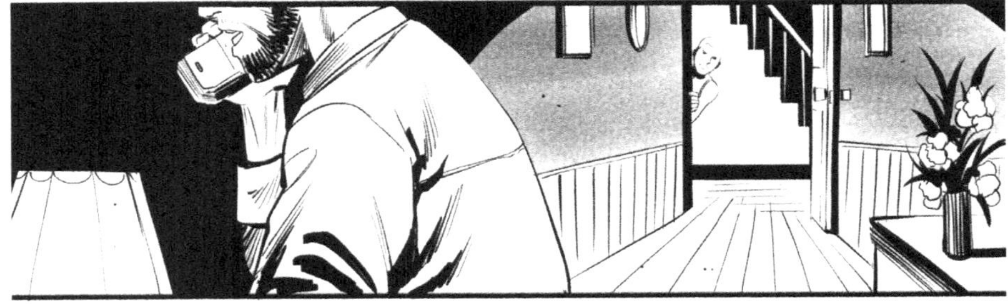
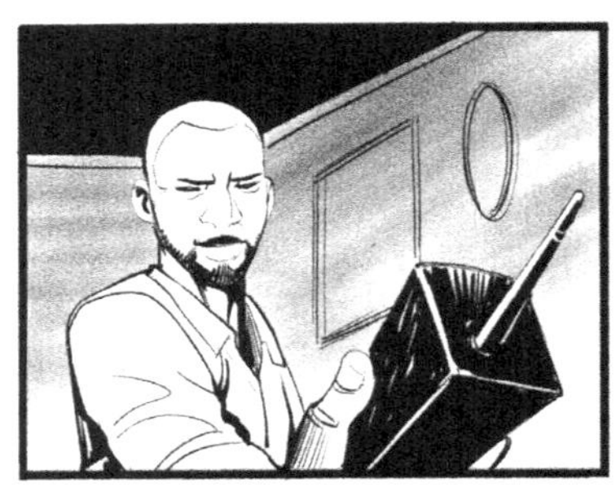
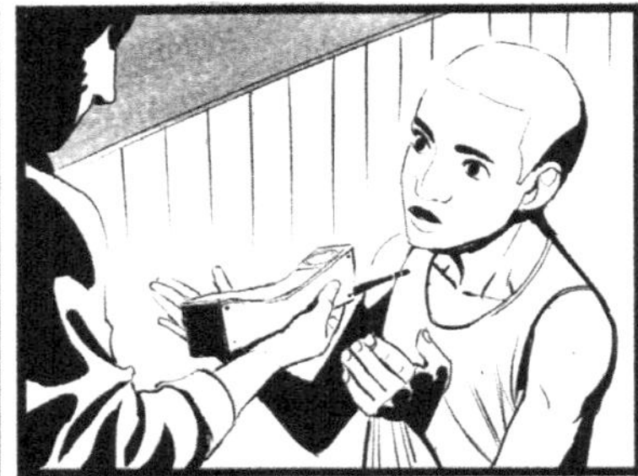
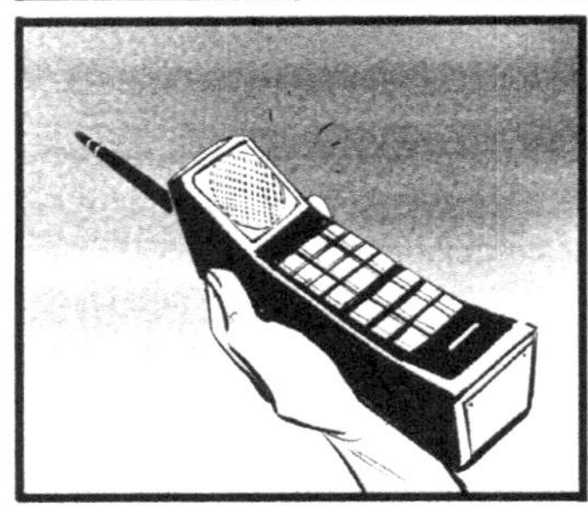
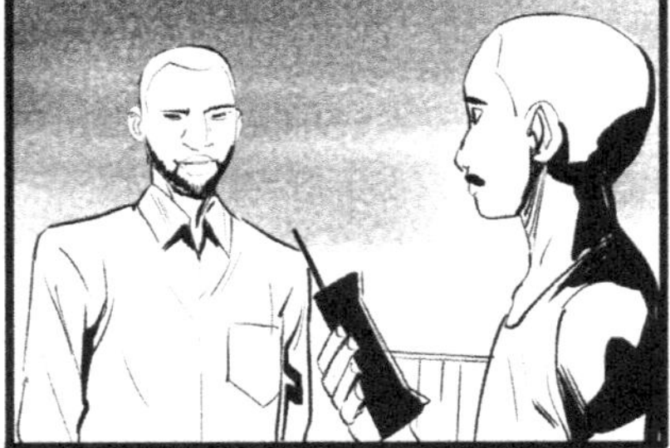

t felt odd sleeping over at my dad's that night. I wanted it to be like this forever, yet there was a lingering voice in the back of my mind that told me not to get too comfortable; this was only temporary. I was restless and my mind was less than peaceful. I wondered if I would have to go back to my abuser's home soon and how long this was going to last. I couldn't go back there. Knowing the feeling of freedom I had now, the sense of peace Dad's home gave me, I knew going back to my abuser's home would break me.

It was Saturday when the phone rang. My dad answered it in the kitchen while I was playing a game in the computer room. When I heard the muffled sound of Her voice through the receiver, my body froze. My dad responded, "Well, you can talk to him if he wants to talk to you."

I hadn't heard from her or seen her in days, but just her voice coming from the other room caused a wave of panic to rumble through my bones, sending a shockwave up my nervous system. Fear overtook me once again. My fingers stopped button mashing the controller and I froze in my chair.

Sitting there, the voices of doubt and fear overtook me momentarily. I didn't want her thinking I didn't want to talk to her anymore, but at the same time I truly didn't want to talk to her. But there was also a part of me that hoped she was somehow changed and wanted to fix everything. At eleven, I was confused and conflicted. So many overwhelming thoughts and emotions were rocketing through me.

I entered the kitchen. He looked at me carefully, seeming to read my thoughts, and then rather than hand me the phone, he put it on speaker.

"H-hello?" I was able to start in a quaky voice.

"Heeeyyy, how are you doing?" she asked excitedly. I couldn't believe how happy she sounded right now.

I asked warily, "I'm ... I'm good ... h-how are you?"

"Good, good! I'm here at a family's football game and ran into a relative who wants to say hey. I'm going to give her the phone!"

She was playing this off. This was all a spectacle. A fake performance. I knew it well. But still, how the heck could she be pretending everything was "normal"? I didn't want to talk to the other person. I didn't want to talk to anyone, but I couldn't just hang up either.

The relative on the other line and I exchanged meaningless pleasantries. I responded with short sentences, more confused than ever. I didn't know why this person sounded so cheerful. What was going on? Why were they so happy? Why did they call my dad's house phone? They never called his house phone.

Did they know something I didn't? Why wasn't this going like I thought it would?

The relative then handed the phone back over to my abuser, and I heard Her voice once again. Chills sprang back up my spine. "Okay, it was good talking to you. I love you!" And then she paused. "I'll see you soon, bye!"

*Click*

What did she mean by that? I looked at Dad with desperation. I looked at him for answers, begging him with my eyes when I asked, "I'm not going back over there Monday, am I?"

Even when he shook his head, there was doubt in my heart. My anxiety was feeding me paranoid thoughts. Did she know something he didn't know? She had talked over the phone as if nothing had changed, so what if nothing really had changed?

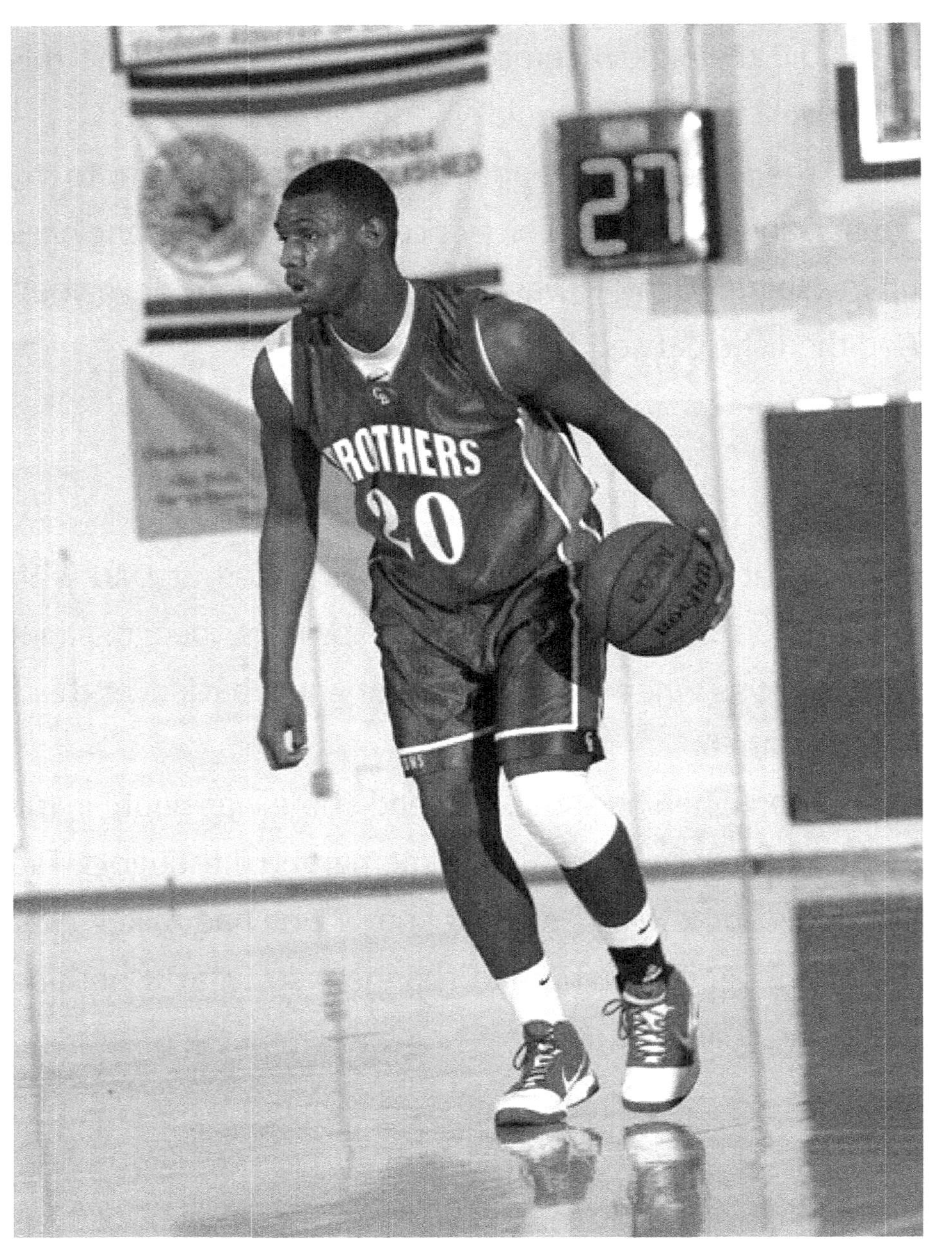

# 27

# INTERNAL VICTORY LEADS TO EXTERNAL SUCCESS

As I mentioned in an earlier chapter, if someone has no self-confidence, it leaves an empty space for something else to fill. So what will fill it?

If we look at my life, the hole that was supposed to hold my confidence and self-worth was filled with mental challenges: depression, anxiety, PTSD, fear, worry, doubt, et cetera. I believe it's the same for other people. The cocktail might be a bit different from person to person, but the destructive forces of the ingredients are the same. If we do not see the value in ourselves, if we don't have confidence to want to grow and have a future, if we do not have the faith and resilience to carry ourselves over the threshold, then sometimes we just never make it to where we wished to be.

Without: (1) self-worth, (2) resilience, and (3) discipline, then we don't achieve those passionate goals. We don't obtain that dream job. We don't get that fateful first date. We don't receive that hopeful scholarship. We just fail. We pour our entire selves into something that's safe or just flat out easy.

Now, why do we fail?

That's a great question. There are many answers to this, so I'm going to only touch on a few. We fail for a few reasons. First, if we don't have self-confidence in who we are or what we're capable of, then we just don't even try. We fail automatically because we don't take the leap of faith to even attempt. We make excuses for why we aren't instead of finding good reasons why we should. We are afraid of the unknown, we are afraid to fail, and in that we inevitably do the thing we're scared to do — fail. Marcus Aurelius once said, "It's not death a man should fear, but he should fear never beginning to live."

Another reason we fail is because we only 'try.' We do it half-heartedly, yet the other half is full of doubt. We make an attempt, but in the back of our minds, we aren't confident. A wise Jedi Master once said: "Do or do not. There is no try." We are afraid. In that effort, we still fail, or we just never finish. If you are trying just to say you tried, you are setting yourself up for a guaranteed loss. Henry Ford said this: "One of the greatest discoveries a man makes, one of his great surprises, is to find he could do what he was afraid he couldn't do."

We also fail because we are so concerned by how people see us and what they think. I get it. Our lives are intertwined with other human beings all the time, and it's hard to ignore them. It can be extremely hard to push off the nay-sayers and doubters. They can plant weeds in our minds by the negative and unsupportive words they say. Our fear is like the water, causing the weeds to grow as we tend to those worries. And before we know it, the seed within us — our hopes, dreams, and aspirations — gets choked out, overwhelmed, and failed before it's even started to grow because we've allowed other people — who don't even get to live *our* life — to stop us from trying.

Another reason we fail: we don't think we're good enough. We don't think we have what it takes to be a great … well, anything. That's just a lie you've heard, and it just replays in the back of your mind. I'm telling you that you *are* good enough. Don't be afraid. Have the courage to be bad at something new. I can pretty much guarantee you that the things you are made to do will not look pretty or feel quite "right" the first time, or maybe even for quite some time! But take heart and have faith in yourself. You do have gifts and talents that you were made for, and when you find them and start to learn them, you'll feel a deep resonance inside you that nothing else quite touches. One day, an opportunity will come, and when you're ready, you'll step through that door with utter confidence.

I remember a quote from Wally Amos: *"Never be afraid of trying something new. Remember, amateurs built the ark; professionals built the Titanic."*

Though there are numerous other reasons for failure, I believe this is another strong reason we fail. We give up too soon. We don't have the patience or discipline or resilience to keep going. The journey to your dream is sort of like the journey to getting a college degree. You start young and you work through steps every year. Each year those steps get harder. But over time, with discipline and patience and faith, you'll achieve that degree. When you started those courses, you weren't ready for the final tests. Learning takes time. Just like there are no shortcuts to graduating college, in the same way there are no shortcuts to achieving your dreams. Admiral William H. McRaven stated, "If you want to change the world, start off by making your bed." Then build on each small accomplishment.

So, don't give up early. Enjoy the ride. Learn on the way. Take each day for what it is — a gift. Each hour is a treasure. Be successful daily in some small way. Learn, learn, learn. Knowledge is invaluable, and you have loads of free access to build that knowledge. Soon, you'll get to your goal. As Thomas Edison said: *"Our greatest weakness lies in giving up. The most certain way to succeed is always to try just one more time."*

If you keep telling yourself 'just go one more day', then you'll soon realize after weeks and months and years of never giving up, you believe it and you won't ever want to quit. The journey through life is too incredible. You are an adventurer on a quest to self-discovery. So, keep putting one foot in front of the other. Erase the doubt and fear inside your mind, and the world will reveal the dream you've worked so hard for.

It took me over twenty years to be an NFL football player. Our friend, Kent Ferguson, the Olympic diver, didn't make the Olympic team until he was 29 years old. I dare you to work just as hard as us for your goal.

# OVERTIME REFLECTION

- What are the toughest challenges you face every day?

- How can your new habits help you get through those challenges?

- Who do you see yourself as 5 years from now?

# 28

# WHAT NEXT?

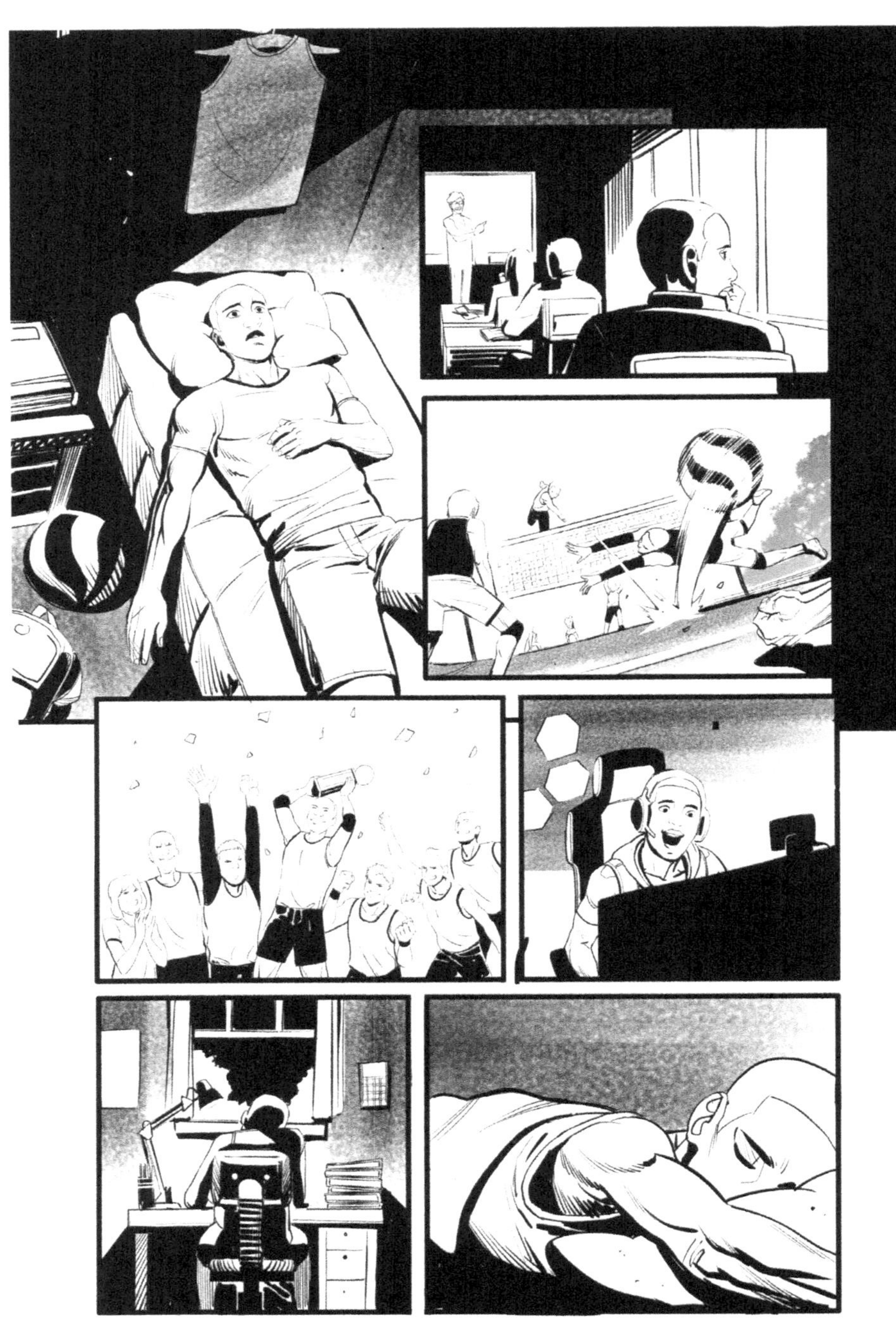

The end of my sixth grade school year was approaching quickly. I was officially living with my dad now, which should have brought me peace, but internally I was a mess. The school I attended was a private school, and was strict about education. Any grades or classes that were performing below a 70% were considered failing, so it was a tough school academically. Typically, I was a Gold Honor Roll student with a GPA of 3.8 or higher.

But as the year was ending, I began to fall apart — emotionally, academically, socially, and mentally. Dad was patient with me. He understood that trauma and anxiety still had a full grip on me, and he was always cool-tempered.

For example, one day he asked me to take out the trash.

I responded coldly. "What if I don't? You gonna hit me?"

He looked at me and blinked; surprised, yet not surprised. "No, I'm not going to hit you, but I will be disappointed."

His response was enough to get me back on track, and there weren't too many more exchanges like this between us. I was subconsciously testing him, but I was learning that he wasn't anything like my abuser. I was also learning that I never wanted to disappoint him. He did so much to keep me safe, so I needed to do what I could to be a better son.

School however, was a different story. I started bombing most of my classes. I couldn't focus and I didn't care about my grades. My mental barriers were difficult to overcome, and my priorities had changed. I wasn't comprehending my work or retaining the information I was learning in class. My 'survivor brain' was still fully operational. Every time I went outside for recess with my friends, my eyes were on the road and parking lot. I felt certain She was watching and waiting for her opportunity to strike. Classes were a haze every day, and it concerned my teachers and father. I started to act out, becoming a class clown instead of a good student.

I finished out my sixth grade year in this fog of anxiety and emotional stew. It wasn't until summertime that I began to finally relax, cope, and adapt. I began to adjust to regular life outside of school. A life not lived in constant fear or watching my back. I began to learn to be calm, have a routine, and healthy interactions with my dad.

Most days I spent with Dad and his future wife. She was amazing. She'd come down on weekends and let us spend the holidays with her side of the family. Her whole family was incredibly welcoming and inviting. They took me in as one of their own, and I'll never forget how that felt. Once Dad married, she truly became Mom. I love her dearly. It was amazing to have these wonderful people in my corner. But my dad, he didn't have much family around. So most of the time, it was just us three. Thanks to all the quality time, we began building an even stronger father-son relationship as well. It meant everything to me and was a lot of fun.

Dad also felt the need to put me in therapy in order to work out any resentment I had towards my abuser, as well as any resentment that I might have developed towards women in general. He was concerned that my abuse would subconsciously force me to perceive women in a different light; in a negative light. Thankfully, I was able to work through those barriers and learn more about myself over time.

Then, near the beginning of my new school year, my father had a meeting with his lawyer. What he told me changed my attitude about my academics. It turned out, when She had found out about my grades dropping, she had been using that as leverage. She had legal rights and was going to use whatever methods she could to get me back in her clutches if possible.

Dad told me I needed to make a choice about how to handle my academics. With those words, I knew I had to do everything in my power to stay where I was. I had to go back to being consciously aware of being a good student. I wasn't going to let Her win. I liked my life now, so I was going to fight for it. The changes in my life so far had happened because I had stood up for myself, so I knew I had to keep making smart choices. I needed to keep growing. No more maintaining or being complacent. If I wanted to keep hope, I had to care.

That next school year — seventh grade — I made an effort to do better. My focus and work-ethic improved. I was able to pay attention in class and demonstrate improved behaviors. There were less concerns and red flags, but teachers still checked in on me. By this point, I had stopped playing soccer and was starting to excel in basketball. I also tried out for the flag football team, which was pretty fun. By the end of the year, I finished with average grades.

The summer was quieter in my heart and mind than the previous year. I hadn't seen my abuser since that last beating a year and a half ago, and I hadn't spoken to her since the strange call at my dad's my first weekend there. I enjoyed the warm, summer months before the next school year. By 8th grade, I really started to grow — physically and emotionally. I had shot up to 6'1". Because of my height, I joined the boys' volleyball team. We dominated the competition, winning the championship that year.

Academically, my mindset stayed on course. I was succeeding, in spite of Her. By 8th grade, the school put me in accelerated classes. I got the best grades I'd ever had in my life. Her attempts to use my academics to manipulate the system would never fly. I was standing up for myself and it felt amazing. I was doing it for me.

Then one day, a friend of mine came to one of my classes. "Asante, I think She's here." This was a friend I had entrusted with the truth about my abuse, so he knew how big of a deal this was for me, and I greatly appreciated it.

I knew exactly who he was talking about, too. "What?"

"Yeah, she's at the front desk."

With an excuse to use the bathroom, I left class and scouted the halls. I tip-toed down past all the classes, cautiously and silently. I peeked around the corner and eyed the office ... there She was, her back to me. I was pretty sure she hadn't seen me. It was the first time I had seen her in over a year, and it churned my guts. I was mad. She didn't need to be here. After a while, I told myself to leave. I didn't need to be here either, so I went back to class, hoping the school was going to keep her away from me. They did.

I knew my dad was still talking to lawyers and going to court later that year, so Her presence at the school had to have meant something. But what? Why was she there?

# 29

# MINDSET AND IDENTITY

Seneca, a Roman philosopher, stated: "*I do not distinguish by the eye, but by the mind, which is the proper judge of the man.*"

There is always a point in our life — at a young age or older — when we ponder the person we are or who we want to become. We typically look backward to see what we've accomplished and how we got here, or we envision our future, often based on people we aspire to be like. But for some of us, looking backward into our lives can be an ugly place to go. It can dredge up regret or shame. It's hard to understand how we're supposed to fit into this big, mysterious world. It's even harder to understand that we can play a beneficial role in it. We may feel like we've already missed our chance. But let me be the first to say, you haven't. If you are alive and breathing, you are *already* making an impact and you have something amazing to offer! It was true for me as well.

Around 8th grade, I started to recognize that I was becoming a 'somebody,' but I wasn't exactly sure who that 'somebody' was supposed to be. I had gotten a taste of my very first championship that year in volleyball. I was also in my second year of flag football, and basketball had become my new favorite sport.

But when I looked around me, I saw that I stood out a bit. Sure, maybe it was because I was already over six feet tall by this point, or maybe it was because I was truly starting to feel like *myself.* It was less about wearing a mask, and more about becoming comfortable in my very own skin ... and letting that 'skin' show. I enjoyed where I was at. Athletically and academically, I was challenging myself. I was feeling good about who I was because I was taking back my own power, and with it my own confidence. I was molding myself into someone I enjoyed being.

So how do we figure out who you are and who you're supposed to be? Well, sometimes it is quite difficult to find out. There are many areas of a person we must look at, and we can start with a simple first question to this little self-assessment. What are your passions and what are your hobbies? This isn't necessarily the answer to your question, but it is a great place to gather clues. From there however, we need to explore the mindset that goes with the pursuit of your interests. You will quickly find that certain areas of interest can have unhealthy mindsets that dominate that field of work.

For example, in this new era of advanced technology, many youth would identify that their future might have to do with becoming a Youtuber or social media influencer. The mindset here can become one of self-absorption and a need for acceptance, or it could be a desire to help other people achieve their own goals and greatness. One has a need to be validated outwardly, and the other already knows they have something worthwhile to offer. The mindset matters *greatly* in the success of your own future.

When looking at our personalized goals and passions, we have to recognize and fine-tune our mindset towards success. If you want to be a professional athlete, you can't neglect your academics, no matter how uninteresting they may be to you. If you want to get into business, you have to learn to understand people and how to treat them well, not just focus on how to get money in your wallet.

Many people want to get to the top in whatever passion they have, but will trample anyone around them to reach their dream. When the mindset becomes "I'll do whatever it takes," no matter the damage done to others, they may reach the mountaintop, but they will find it to be a cold and lonely place.

Mindset will make all the difference in how you reach those goals while being the best you can be in this world. You have amazing things to offer.

There are also some of us who have no idea yet who they are or what they want to do in the future. That's okay too, but I personally encourage you to at least *think* about what you might want to do with your life before college or before you start a career. It's okay to acknowledge you are still learning to find yourself. But don't be afraid to just try something. It may lead to new passions you never even knew existed! The only guaranteed way to fail is to never try.

Even if you don't know exactly what you want to do or what you want to accomplish, just use your time building your knowledge and identifying the natural skills you have or skills you want to have that help you make an impact. We *all* have different talents and abilities for different reasons.

So, why are millions of Americans so unhappy with the type of work they do? Why do so many people go to their job day in and day out, but are depressed? Why aren't people doing what they absolutely love doing? These are the right questions because maybe it will help us understand where you want to be in a decade.

In this life, we get one chance to fulfill that destiny that lies inside of us. I was destined to be a football player for a time, but what if I had chosen the route of a businessman instead? Yes, I would have worked very hard at my job, because I know the value of hard work, but I don't believe I would have been satisfied with that type of career. Even if it had made me a phenomenally wealthy businessman, I *still* don't think I'd actually be happy. Why?

Because football was my heart. I put a decade of

passion into athletic competition. I was disciplined to compete and determined to grow physically and mentally. Had I cut all that out in an instant to be a businessman, it wouldn't have resonated with my spirit. It wouldn't have fueled me. I wasn't doing what I was meant to do. It wouldn't have fit what I was destined to do at the time.

Some of you may be a bit skeptical about the 'destined for' talk we're currently having, so let me help you understand where I'm coming from. Every single human being is born different — Yes, including identical twins. We have similarities here and there, but internally we are nothing alike. And I'm not talking just about physical characteristics. Think about it — billions of different individuals with different skills and different circumstances and different dreams. I'm also talking about what's on the inside; in the mind and in the heart. These are the places of a person we don't spend a lot of time looking at.

Now, let's exclude life circumstances just for a moment and reflect on all the other realms of what makes our character or identity. This world offers many forms of entertainment, knowledge, hobbies, skills, outlets, and interests. There are so many different things that draw us in — fame and celebrity life, different parts of the world, movies, books, academic courses, theatre, the Arts, colors, foods, passions, holidays, culture, history, science, the stars, and the list goes on. People respond (or resonate) differently to these things.

I enjoy going to the gym, but I know there are many people who can't stand it. There are people who enjoy socializing with other people and people who avoid human interaction entirely. There are people who love animals more than humans, and there are people who understand *things* more than people. There are people who enjoy exploring the mysteries of the world, while others prefer exploring the digital world of coding and programming from their home or cubical. Some thrive off competition, others love to cook. Some want to perfect something already made, while others spend their life inventing something new. Some people like to act, others like to write. Some people prefer singing, others prefer dancing. Some have a passion to speak to an audience, others have a passion to work one-on-one. Some want to be defenders of children, while others want to understand how to fight away cancers and diseases. Some want to be soldiers while others want to do missionary work in third-world countries. And this list goes on forever and ever. The point is, something is meant for *all* of us, yet there is a specific set of giftings that fits us perfectly. And those gifts are something you could do the rest of your life, for free if you had to. That's destiny.

So the next question is: who are you meant to be?

And that's the right question, but to get to that answer we have to ask many other questions. I cannot have the direct answer for you, because we're searching out *your* destiny. What I can offer, however, is the story of how I found my own.

# OVERTIME REFLECTION

- What obstacles stand between you and your future self?

- How do you plan to overcome those obstacles, and are you willing to start now?

- Who do you want to be in ten years?

# 30

# UNVEILING YOUR HIDDEN GIFT

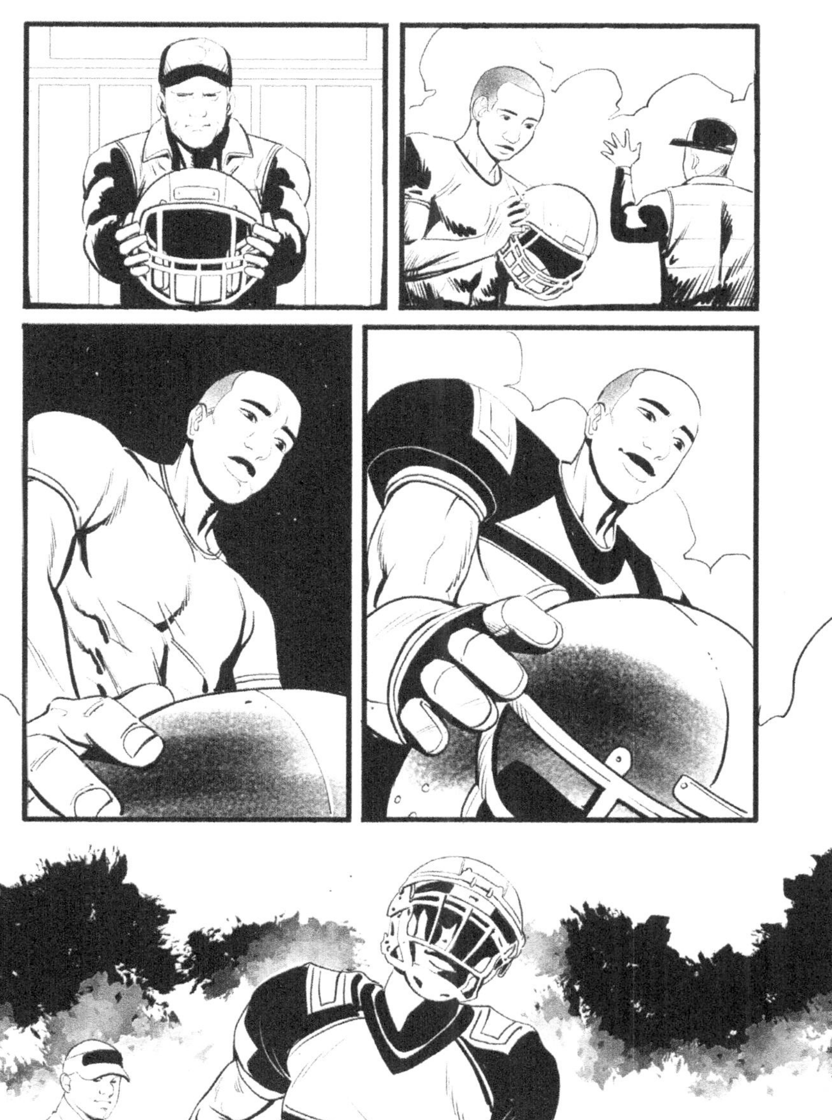

fter the unnerving sighting of my abuser in the school office, I didn't see her again. My summer before freshman year started was great. I was so excited to see what high school had to offer. There were going to be upperclassmen, girls, sports, and new classes with a whole lot of familiar and unfamiliar faces. Then right before school started, something unexpected happened. I grew another 3 inches. I was now 6'4".

During freshman orientation, a football coach approached me and asked if I wanted to try out for the football team. I didn't see why not. I was already one of the best and tallest basketball players. I felt this would be my in to make a name for myself in high school. Adjusting to the new school environment wasn't too hard for me academically, but it was socially. I was a middle-of-the-pack kind of student. But if I wanted to make a name for myself, being that I was so competitive, then I knew sports was the way.

The coach confidently said I would be perfect for football, so if it was anything like 8th grade volleyball, then I had another chance to bring home a championship for my school, but this time it was *high* school. I had hopes that football would come as naturally to me as basketball, volleyball, and soccer had.

When I got to my very first football practice, they asked me what position I wanted to play. I told them I wanted to be a wide receiver. It wasn't just because I wanted to catch the football and make epic plays. It was because I wanted to score touchdowns while doing it. I wanted to be like all the other great receivers I watched on TV. Plus, I figured people loved watching the impact players or play-makers more than anyone else, so yeah … I went with the wide receiver.

Well, I hadn't even made it out of football camp before I was 'demoted' to tight end. This was a huge bummer for me because I felt this new position was a slap in the face. Despite my desire to be great, I still wasn't a confident athlete. If I was naturally good at something and didn't have to compete to be the best, then I was satisfied. But, when they pulled me from the routes and placed me on the line, it really gutted me. I felt like I wasn't good enough at being a wide receiver, and I took the new position as a way of them saying, "Let's just put Asante over here. Keep him outta the way."

For the rest of the football season, we did okay. As a team we weren't great or the best, nor was I a stand-out player. There were a few brief moments where my talent showed on the field, but nothing that made it to the highlight reel. To me, it didn't seem football was all that it was cracked up to be. I wanted to be done with it entirely. It was too hard, painful, and required so much work to improve. I didn't think I wanted to go out for the team the next year. And to prove that I was hesitant to do another year of football, I went out for Track & Field spring season to skip football training. I chose to do shotput and discus instead. Less work and an easier way to avoid spring training.

Sophomore year was the year I almost completely threw in the towel for football. I was debating walking into Coach's office and quitting. In fact, my dad almost did the quitting for me, but after talking to a couple friends, I realized I still wanted to see what I could do on the field. I had to prove to myself that football was, in fact, *not* what I wanted to do. I needed to try one more time, with last year's experience under my belt.

Stepping out onto the field for football camp sophomore season, I was shocked to learn many of my previous year's teammates had quit — just like I had planned. And by the end of football camp, almost 50% of the guys were done with the sport, leaving only around 25 athletes left playing.

But let me tell you, this group of guys that stuck it out ended up being extremely committed to each other and to succeeding. We formed a bond, a tight-knit relationship, with each other because we shared a similar mindset. We were like a hive-mind, doing everything we could to take care of each other and our responsibilities on the field. We worked well together because we all had a passion for the sport. We wanted to see what we could do after a 'so-so' freshman season. Most of that wouldn't have happened had it not been for the coaching staff. They challenged and pushed us, but also guided and supported us. They helped us believe in ourselves, and they inspired us to give them our hearts. Together, we had confidence that we were a really good team. And we were. Our season ended with nine wins and only one loss.

That year, we won the Holy Bowl, which was one of the oldest rivalry games in California history. Even though we were just the Junior Varsity team, it didn't matter. We had done something amazing for our school, and it gave us the confidence to set a huge goal — to win this bowl game as seniors, something our school hadn't done for eight years. It would be a game to remember — playing our rivals, Jesuit High School, in front of 17,000 fans.

Even though I still classified myself as a basketball player, I was seeing myself in a different light because of football. The tight end position required blocking, catching, and running — a trifecta of skills and talents that required more time to master. It was a challenge, but there was no way I was going to run away from that challenge now that I was fitting into something special. These guys depended on me, and I was learning a lot more about myself in this position.

I learned to *love* being a tight end. I learned to respect it, not because it was a job, but because it was *my* job. I wasn't going to be mopey about it any longer. And I fell in love with it more and more the harder I worked at it. Besides, they fed me the ball like crazy in that position. Not only did I catch the ball, run with the ball, and score touchdowns, but I also got to block alongside the linemen, a football position that had all the guts yet received none of the glory.

After football season, I realized sports were really my jam. I was the only sophomore who started on the Varsity basketball team. It was still the sport I believed that would get me to college. But the more I focused on sports, the more my grades began to slip. I became content with putting all my focus into my sports instead of into my education. I lost my balance. I started getting distracted. And in the next year or two, I was going to see the results of those mistakes.

# 31

# TAKE THE WHOLE LEMON TREE

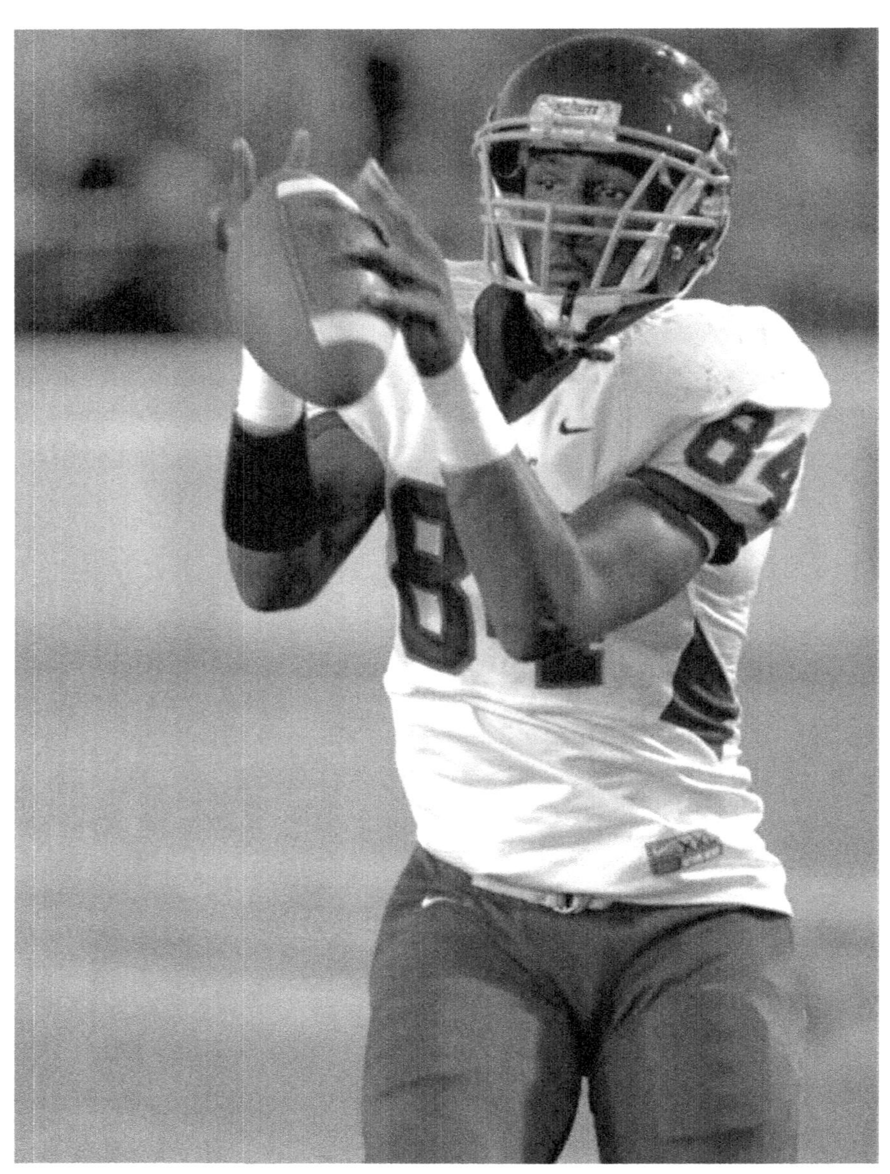

You know the proverbial phrase, "When life gives you lemons, make lemonade?" I really like what it's trying to tell us — make something good out of something bad. And I believe that statement rings true to many people, but I also feel that there are people in this world who feel life's not handing them those lemons, it's bombarding them with an endless lemon assault!

There are so many incredible people on this planet who can't catch a break. Their life is constantly overwhelmed with 'lemons,' and their chances for a future seem hopeless. I get it. I've been through it. So, let's reword this proverbial phrase one more time: "When life gives you lemons, don't just make lemonade. Take the whole freakin' lemon tree."

Find the source of the lemons (your life) and take control of it. Don't be content with the bitterness of your life, nor be content with the sweetness you may make of some of it. Take advantage of learning about your world, the one that surrounds you, and adjust to it consciously. Be deliberate with how you must adjust to the hand you've been dealt. Make a stronger one, one that fits you right.

What do we need to know in order to make this change? Again it comes back around to mindset. It's the gears we put ourselves in when we coast down the freeway of life. What kind of mindset do you currently carry around with you? Optimism or pessimism? Dramatic or self-aware? Positive or negative? Kind or selfish? Fake or real? Attention-seeking or attentive? Do some mind-searching and figure out how you want to impact the world online or in the social environment.

Next, we must be honest with ourselves when assessing how we handle the distractions that can consume us; that can take us away from our future goals. Currently, with social media being such a distracting piece of entertainment, there is a big concern about how it is becoming the 'New World' of how people live. We use it in our daily conversations, we use it to assess ourselves based on others, we use it as a way to create different identities, we use it to learn about others by avoiding social interactions with them, we use it to influence/be influenced, and we use it to cope. Now, I'm not saying social media or electronic devices are a bad thing — I enjoy video games and social media as a tool I use to connect with people. But, *too* much can be unhealthy, chemically, mentally, and emotionally.

Too much exposure causes our brain to go in 'robot mode,' where it's hard to transition back to the conscious part of our brain. This makes learning and processing new information more of a challenge. And the conscious (or aware) part of our brain is where we need to make direct, deliberate decisions every day towards what we were created to do in this world.

Then factor in the changes in the world that began during 2020. School and in-person interactions got even more limited, so that greatly increased this method of socialization and communication and even education.

So, how much of it do you fill your brain with? Is the information useful or useless? Are these hours being spent wisely or are they wasted?

What we're looking for in ourselves is found on a journey of self-discovery. Very little useful information about yourself can be found looking at a screen. Our bodies were meant to move and interact with the world around us! I found it was much more enjoyable *being* on the football field rather than watching the game from my living room. So let's get into figuring out the gloves that fit. I encourage you to stop here for a second and grab a paper and pen as you answer these questions. These kinds of things are even more helpful when you can see them in black and white, and be able to refer to them over and over as needed.

## What You've Got to Work With

1. *What is something you're good at that comes to you naturally?*

I think this is a solid foundational question we can start at. Are you a people-person? What classes do you always look forward to in school? Are fabrics and clothing design something you always think about? Are paints and canvases your best friend? Do you have an eye for beauty, nature, and the world? Can you carry or dribble a ball in your sleep? Can you carry a tune, and do you sing more than you talk? Do numbers and equations come to you easily? Could you escape into stories just as quickly as one can escape into an acting role? These are just a few examples of questions worth reflecting on when answering the first question. Don't worry about if it's something you can make a "job" from, just write out things you know you're good at.

Some may say that they have a variety of talents, or that they're able to do many different things naturally. Remember the saying, "Jack of all trades, master of none, though ofttimes better than master of one." It's good to have many talents, but don't let yourself get comfortable with being mediocre at many talents. Improve on as many of them as possible.

2. *What are some skills and talents you know you don't have?*

Not everyone can sing well, which is alright. I can't sing at all. Some people are terrible with mechanical work.

I know nothing about mechanical work. Others are just terrible with understanding people. Some people can't draw much better than a stick-figure portrait. There are some people who aren't good at running heavy machinery or working in a kitchen. What I'm saying is that it's okay to *not* be great at something. We're all *not* good at something in some aspect in our life. Just assess yourself honestly, but be kind to yourself. This isn't a list of failures, just *non-skills*.

3. *What skills and talents do you <u>want</u> to be good at?*

Football didn't come naturally to me, but it was something I enjoyed and that I wanted to perfect, so I had to work at it. Some people want to learn to be a pilot, and that's something that requires lessons. Some people want to act, but don't have the tools *yet* to be a good actor. Some people want to get into public speaking, but their barrier is either dealing with the fear of public speaking or struggling to conjure up sentences and words that express their hearts and thoughts. Heck, some of your non-skills may even fall into this category. That's ok, write them down! Maybe you're only bad at it now because you haven't had the right teacher. We'll explore that more.

Once you have those three lists written down (natural talents, non-talents, want-to-have-skills), then let's move on to the next topic.

## Motivation

1. *What fills you with nearly limitless energy?*

Have you ever talked to a photographer or a painter or a graphic designer? They have such a unique mindset on how they perceive the world around them. If there's a local business with a bad logo, they'll say something. If the sun catches the horizon just right, they'll take a billion pictures just for that one perfect shot. If there is a napkin in front of them, they'll start doodling. It's amazing, because it's something they'll do for free for the rest of their lives. Why? It *energizes* them, almost like a dose of a superpower. So, what fills you with energy?

As an athlete, I loved strapping on those shoulder pads. I looked forward to the challenging workouts in the gym. I enjoyed throwing on my jersey and stepping out onto the field. I loved how it felt to try to be the best at what I do. I knew I could help people feel energized and filled with passion when they watched me play. It was something I was willing to do for free for the rest of my life if I had to.

Take your time with this question. It's important to recognize what those one or two or three things are that really resonate with you. After you're done, let's move on to the third topic.

## Interests

1. *What draws in your focus?*

This could be something you can't stop talking or thinking about. This could be something you bug your family or friends about often at home or school. This could be a class where the teacher influences you to improve because the material you're studying draws you in daily. This could be a genre of books you enjoy reading. It could even be a specific piece of history at a museum that keeps you mesmerized. Maybe you're obsessed with creating new ideas or storylines. It could even be you in your room taking things apart to see how they work, and then putting them back together. What this question is looking for is that "something" you could spend hours doing without knowing you've been spending hours doing it.

If you really aren't sure about these answers, or if you just want to broaden your answers even further, ask someone who really knows you well what they see in you. Often, other people can see things you didn't notice yet. They may recognize potential or inspire things in you that are yet to be fully tapped into. People who truly listen to what you have to say or pay attention to how you respond and behave are likely to have great insight into some of your potential.

After you have answered these questions, don't

throw the list away. Next, we'll be focusing on how to identify short-term and long-term goals, how to hone in your skills towards your goals, and how to take it one step further, one step at a time. If planning out goals isn't your cup of tea, make good habits in the direction that interests you. It's easier to stay where you are, but you'll never get where you want to go.

Are you willing to be patient, to work hard, and to fail numerous times before finally getting what you've dreamt of? Are you willing to go through a five-year, ten-year, twenty-year quest to discover your path and the reason why you were put on this Earth? Are you willing to take risks and make mistakes along the way? I hope so. Because once you have reached the stars, you'll do whatever it takes to stay there. You're worth it and I can't wait to see what you have to offer the world.

# OVERTIME REFLECTION

- Did you do the questions in this chapter? If not, what's holding you back?

- What did you learn about yourself in the process of writing things out?

- How will you apply what you've learned going forward?

# 32

# MISTAKES WERE MADE

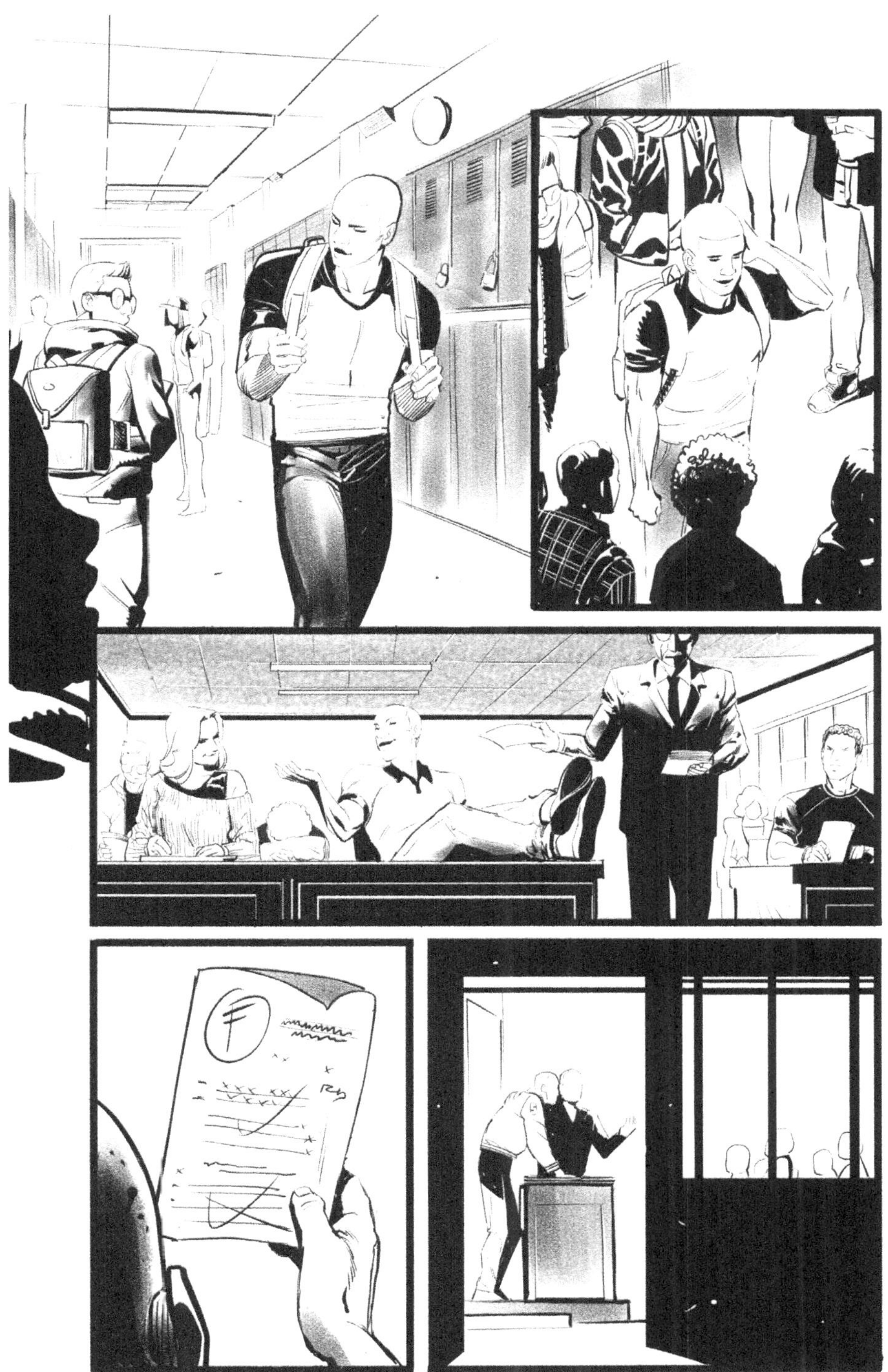

My junior year was a wakeup call for me. It was a great year for football, but because of the reputation I earned, I became distracted and consumed by it. Those distractions took my attention off an important factor of my future — my education. My grades started to drop as I put all my attention into football, basketball, girls, and my social life. One of my closest friends had a car, so we were out driving as much as we were able.

It was intoxicating to be so popular. People knew who I was, and because I was still emotionally starved for positive attention, I soaked it up. I let it take my mind off the things that mattered. I put people around me that pulled me away from my goals and successes. This reckless and distracted mindset was leading me towards some painful life lessons.

The NCAA clearinghouse — where you would register as a student-athlete to be recruited — had a certain GPA requirement, and I was flirting with it. During the football season, my overall GPA dropped half a point from what it was originally, which was around a 2.5.

That was a big deal for me, because I used to be a phenomenal student, but I became complacent, which is poison for the mind and soul, and I didn't care enough to work harder. I maintained decent grades, but the NCAA wasn't looking for decent, they demanded the best from their student-athletes. A good student-athlete was someone who proved they could self-manage, be responsible, be educated, and be trusted. I didn't understand why academics mattered. I just wanted to play football. I wasn't giving my best in the classroom. I became one of those athletes that focused on my sports and my reputation, and in doing so, I failed this particular life challenge.

One day, during the spring, Stanford University coaches came by the school for recruiting. I was one of the athletes they were looking at. Being a naturally academic kid, Stanford would have been the best thing for me. It would have gotten me to places I had always dreamed. I mean, come on … it's Stanford.

But, when they saw my grades, I never got a call back from them, not a single response. I had no one to blame but myself. It was my grades they looked at, not just what I could do on the football field. That was the mistake. That was the fruit of my labor. My ego had won out over my wisdom and I'd only put in half the work. Life gave me a bitter lemon that day. And it really brought me back to reality. What I had done was given up on myself academically. I had betrayed myself, and before I knew it the opportunity I should have been ready for had slipped through my fingers. The door to

Stanford had shut in my face and would never open again. It was disappointing. I didn't stand up for myself and take on the academic challenges in front of me. I neglected some of my gifts, and that was the outcome.

But, the rest of the spring and summer gave me time to process and think. I couldn't allow myself to be defeated. I had to make a choice — stay knocked down or get back up. So I got back up and went to work, harder this time. I finished the school year with a 3.0, and I received my first offer of a full scholarship from the University of Nevada, Reno.

Something around this time had clicked for me. I was so disappointed about Stanford University turning me down, but why? That was the right question. It wasn't just about being disappointed in myself. I was starting to realize that maybe football was something I was *meant* to do. Maybe being a football player was who I was supposed to be. I was starting to get recognized more and more for my athleticism as a football player, but I wasn't getting *any* looks as a basketball player. I had to make another choice — stick with what was getting recognition or keep going the basketball route. If my coaches, fans, peers, and recruiters saw such a potential in me, then this was a point in my life where I had to take a leap of faith and choose a path that I never originally planned to take. I still wasn't fully confident in who I was at this point. But Stanford was a wakeup call, so the right question would be: was I going to answer?

# 33

# LET FAILURE TEACH YOU

When we look at how failure served me up a platter of regret with a side of shame, I want to address that the failure was *not* the point when Stanford University closed the door on me. No, no, no. That was just the fruit of my failure. I didn't put in the labor academically, so all I harvested from it was a missed opportunity.

The failure was actually the slowly built-up bad habits I started creating in the classroom and off the field. Every day that I chose *not* to work hard in my studies, I was failing to tend to the garden I hoped to eat from someday. I put myself in a position where my reputation for sports became a distraction from what mattered most. I put my future on the line while obsessing over praise from people who weren't going to get me to my future goals.

It was ok for me to feel good about others' appreciation. That by itself wasn't a bad thing, but too much of it became academically dangerous for my future. I wasn't balanced.

We need to take credit for what we do well and for what we don't do well, and for me, that included the drop in my GPA, missing Stanford, and the emotional baggage that came with. I only strengthened one leg (sports) over the other leg (academics), and when push came to shove,

I had hindered my ability to move forward in the direction I wanted to go.

So maybe some of you reading this have been knocked off your feet and haven't gotten back up again yet. I get that feeling of wanting to curl up in a ball and cry, or just flat out give up on your dream entirely. It's okay to sit in the struggle for a short while and process through. But I don't want you to stay down there. It won't make things better. If you have a dream or goal, but you feel you fell short, then don't let failure be the answer. Let it be a teacher. Learn from the mistakes you made or from the experience of your circumstances. Consider this moment to be me reaching down and grabbing your hand and pulling you back up onto your feet. It's time to dust off the dirt and get back into the game.

We have a choice on how to respond towards failures. We can either let them remain as failures for the rest of our lives, or we can turn them into a lesson. If you are able to do the latter, then it is no longer classified as failure but renamed a mistake. A mistake is defined as a wrong or misguided action. Once you're aware of it, you know how to avoid it the next time it comes around. You don't have to make the same mistake twice. True failure is making the same mistakes over and over without ever truly learning. One option is a miscalculated misdirection, where you can wander back onto the right path. The other is a guaranteed outcome in the wrong direction. Which would you prefer?

My mistake was taking my eyes off my dreams. When we look at the word 'student-athlete,' we see that there is a hyphen between 'student' and 'athlete.' They are bonded together by that little line. If you want sports and education, then this is your label; this is part of your identity. It's important to give each of them equal attention. Why? That's the right question. As I mentioned before, Stanford wanted an athlete that was responsible, educated, and able to focus their mind *and* body on things that mattered. That's true for other colleges as well. And then there's life after sports. I'll be straight up with you. Being an athlete is something you can do for only a certain amount of years before the body wears out.

I mean, the average age for retiring professional athletes is around 28. Now, I know to you reading this book, 28 years old sounds more like a 105 years old, but 28 catches up to you quickly. Sports isn't something you can do for your entire working life. And sometimes you don't even get to play that long. No one wants to consider the possibility of the unexpected, career-ending injury, but that's exactly what happened to me. Right now, I'm not even thirty years old. I expected to have years ahead of me still on the field, but because I took the time to focus on my education, it has allowed me another path after my career as an NFL athlete ended. My body gave out before my mind did. If I hadn't made the academic changes I did all those years ago, I would have been left with nothing much to work with. What seemed pointless at the time to me, has turned out to be a worthwhile effort after all. Injuries like mine have happened to millions of athletes, to teenagers with dreams. All too often, things don't go as planned. So, then what?

That's a good question, and I'll get to that in later chapters, but for now let's focus on the point of this chapter. Don't ever sell yourself short. You owe yourself the best effort you can perform on and off the field, even if you can't see all the reasons why yet. If you have the opportunity to be challenged in sports, school, the workplace, or even relationships, then face that challenge, overcome it, and learn from it. That's how we grow; through experience and struggle.

# OVERTIME REFLECTION

- On a personal level, does failure help you grow or tempt you to quit?

- Do you take time to reflect on past failures in a positive way? If so, what have you discovered?

- What does it mean to fail, and do you think failure defines you?

# 34

# STOP SECOND GUESSING

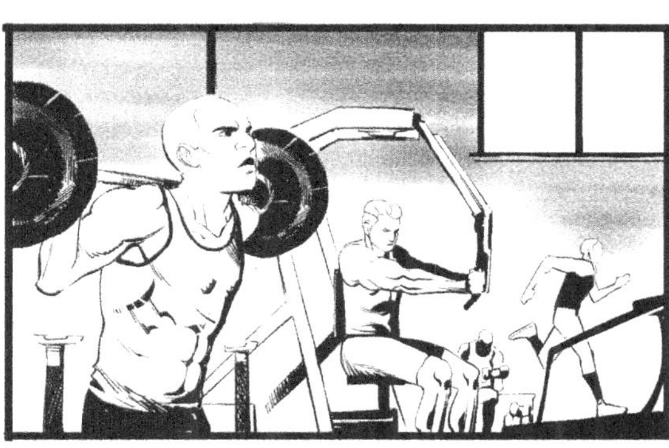
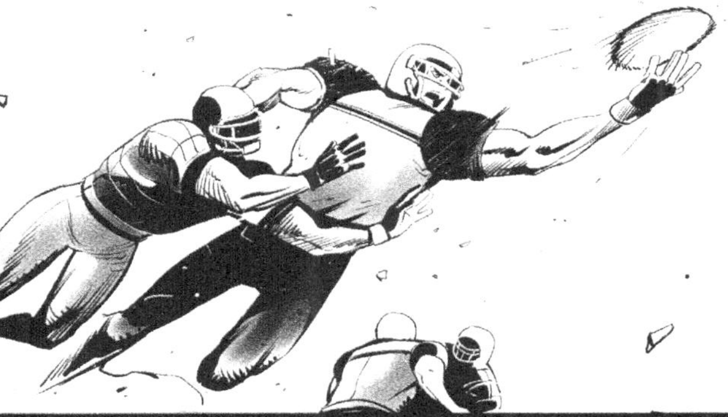
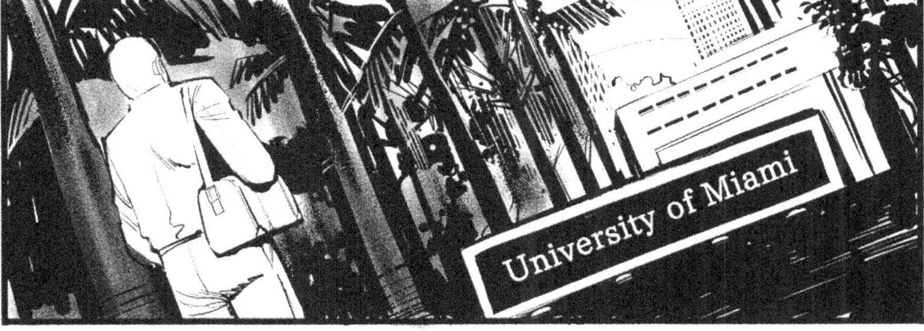
University of Miami
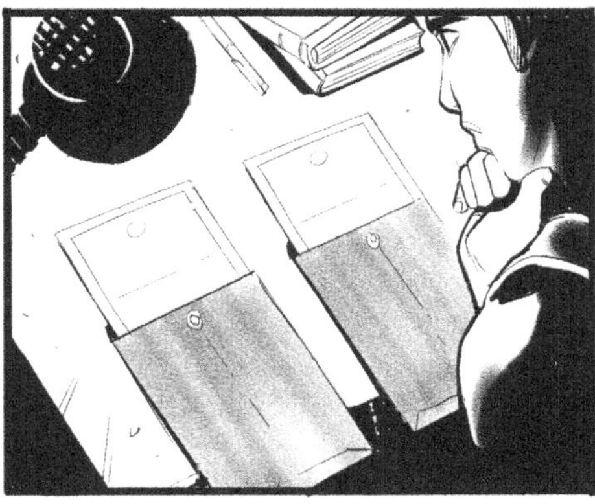
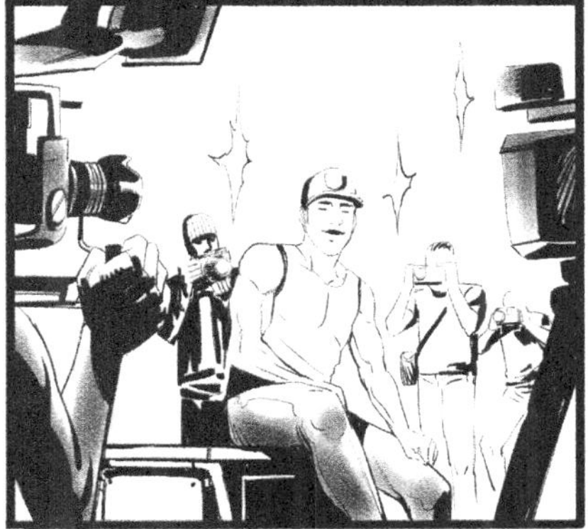

By my senior year, my grade point average had jumped to a 3.3. I didn't want my grades to be a problem ever again when it came to recruitment. I also put more focus and time into my physical training. I had gained over ten pounds of muscle from the start of my junior season to my senior season, now weighing a solid 235 pounds at seventeen years old. I was taking responsibility for being a student and an athlete, yet there was still a part of me that just wasn't confident that I was good enough to take the path of football.

By the end of our senior season, we achieved our goal and won the Holy Bowl against our rivals. This was the first time the varsity team had won the rivalry game in ten years. It felt incredible to be playing with an amazing team that could win it for our school. I was awarded the Great Rivalry Hall of Fame that year, ending the season with 25 catches and over four hundred yards. But much of the attention I received from colleges was because of my blocking capability, not just my catching.

Every play, I dominated my responsibilities until the referee blew the whistle. I showed my grit and my commitment to the team and my position, and this turned heads. Recruiters wanted what I had in their college football programs, but I'd already committed to Washington State

University before the season started. I had wanted to commit early so I could just focus on playing. It had seemed like the best option and best school from all the other offers I had received.

Another influential moment occurred my senior year. I had spent some time studying the rankings of the top tight ends in the country. I wanted to see what they did to get rated so high. I found myself ranked #63 overall going into my senior year, which wasn't too bad, but then I saw a name I was familiar with. There was a guy from another school I had met in summer football camp; he was ranked #37 in the nation. I was shocked to see him rated better than me! At camp I had seen what he could do, and I knew I was better. I was confident I was more talented than him.

And then it hit me, a realization I had never had before. If I was better than this guy, then that meant I was better than most of the others, too. It wasn't ego, it was a simple fact. I had to stop second-guessing who I was on the field because my ranking didn't reflect my athleticism, only my mediocrity. So, I made the decision to go after it, to better my rank. I started the summer workouts off with a new focus and intensity. A couple of my other teammates, who had hopes of playing in college, would work out in the morning with me and one of our coaches. Coach Wiley, who had played in college and the NFL, put us through drills and conditioning, helping us improve our skills. After those workouts, we would still have the team workouts later in the day. (By the way, every person who was in that early morning workout group went on to play in college.)

By the end of the season, my ranking still hadn't changed. My pride was hurt, but when I looked at the big picture, I was still getting attention from D-1 colleges. And I was confident that my stats and hard work deserved better than the rank I still had. This change in me wasn't just about my ranking, but about that little boy all those years ago who had never thought himself to be worthy of greatness, who never thought he was good enough. I had to continue to prove I *was* good enough. I wasn't going to second-guess my talents and abilities. Meanwhile, I had a direction for college, my grades were on point, and my team finished an outstanding varsity season. Things were looking positive, but it wasn't enough for me.

Then one day, my friend Eddie helped me make a highlight tape filled with short clips of my top plays, blocks, and catches I had made throughout the season. I thought it was pretty good, but many people thought it was more than that. Since I had already made a verbal commitment to a college, I wasn't putting much thought into what this could do for me. I was just enjoying having some of my best work showcased, but surprisingly, the highlight tape actually moved my ranking up! I was now #14 best tight end in the country ... all thanks to Eddie and the video we had made.

Less than a week later, my dad was driving me home from school when he casually said, "University of Miami is trying to get a hold of you." He was so nonchalant, I wasn't sure I'd heard right, but it turned out my friend's dad knew a guy who was best friends with the head coach of the University of Miami football team. The head coach had seen my highlight tape and somehow networked his way back down to my dad. The coach had loved the tape and wanted to meet me ASAP because it was the end of recruiting season. I told him I had already made a verbal commitment to Washington State University, but he didn't mind. He just wanted a little bit of my time to talk.

Two days later, the coach called me and offered a full scholarship to the University of Miami. I hadn't expected this. The news was amazing, but I was conflicted. I had made a verbal commitment to another college, and I didn't want to break my word with that football program. So, the coach brought me out to Miami for a visit. The entire time leading up to the trip, I studied the pros and cons between the two colleges. Both academically and athletically, University of Miami was the better choice. It was in the top fifty best schools, but again I was still conflicted.

The tour of the school was incredible. I felt strongly that this was the place for me. Meanwhile, the coaching staff of Washington State had gotten word that I was visiting another school, so they were calling me left and right. I never answered because I knew it was important to hone in on *my* future choices. The first day back after the visit, the coaches from Washington State University were at my school, talking themselves up and talking the other school down.

I knew where I *wanted* to go. My heart said University of Miami, but the voices in my head were telling me to stick with my verbal commitment to Washington State University to be a man of my word. While all of this was going on, the pressure about my decision was high. Friends at school were asking me where I was going. It brought me loads of stress and endless nights of sleeplessness. I struggled to focus, and everywhere I went, people wanted to know which school I wanted to pick. Only two people knew where I wanted to go, but I was struggling to understand what the right choice was.

Then, another moment of clarity hit me. The coaches at Washington State University were pressuring me to keep my commitment, but they were asking something of me that they wouldn't have even asked of themselves. Coaches moved on from programs all the time if it wasn't what they wanted, why should I be held to a higher standard? I realized these men didn't care about what was best for *me*, they cared about what they wanted for the school.

I was tired of second-guessing myself, and I was done holding to other people's expectations of me. I was starting to recognize my mind was full of a lot of lies that I had believed for too long. I needed to just cut everyone's opinions out for now, and listen to my own. I knew where I wanted to go, and I needed to do what was best for me, because this was *my* future and the path that was laid out for me. No one else.

My school counselor helped formulate the appropriate words for my speech on the day of my announcement, but she also encouraged me to use my own words to express myself as well. I committed and signed with the University of Miami. This was an unexpected door that had been opened to me, and I had spent many hours thinking about my decision. I wasn't looking for other people's appreciation, opinions, or approval like I had done for many years before. I took personal responsibility for this decision, and I was proud of myself for it.

I was finally becoming my own man. I was being the person I needed to be for my future. I was finding myself and my purpose in the world. It was an important moment in my life, because two weeks later, I was going to have to face my abuser once again … this time in court.

# 35

# DON'T LISTEN TO THE LIES

As important as good choices, good habits, self-confidence, self-worth, discipline, learning from our mistakes, and resilience are, we also need to deal with the lies we are told and the lies we hear in our society and most importantly, the lies we believe.

I know each of us were gifted with a very specific set of talents and skills that our minds, bodies, and hearts were meant to fulfill in our world. We all feel success in a very individualized way. We also filter the world and perceive things in our own ways, so there may be many things we believe that, in actuality, are not true.

I want to go over a few lies that dogged me as a child and all the way through college and why these lies work against our success, goals, hopes, and dreams. But I'm also going to address the counter-effect lies that we may have told *ourselves* for years. These counter-effect lies are untruths that *sound* like they will be helpful, but aren't. Confusion about what to believe often causes us to hesitate to take the steps we *need* to take towards our goals. So, let's go crush these lies and get after our destiny, yeah?

**Lie #1** — You're Not Good Enough ... But You Can Be

Anything You Want to Be

How many times have you told yourself that you aren't good enough for something, yet society is telling you that you can be anything you want to be? How many times have you thought a challenge was too great or a hope was too big, yet we hear society tell you that your dreams are just a click away or at a certain college? How many times have you compared yourself to influencers on social media or successful entrepreneurs you see on Youtube? How do we know which one is the truth? That's the right question! The truth can't be found in either version. Both of these lies are devastating statements that plant bad seeds in our minds. These lies feed off one another, becoming bigger and bigger the more we think about it.

Imagine each person as a beautiful garden. Everyone's will look different, with a few basic similarities. Now imagine that as life brings some good circumstances, little flowers pop up all around. Peace and beauty reign. But then there are times where bad things in our lives happen, and that's when weeds start to pop up. The harder life gets, the more weeds there are. And if we aren't paying attention, those weeds will grow deep roots and begin to spread.

If weeds aren't plucked, they spread, right? Well, these lies we are discussing are  those weeds, and we need to figure out how to uproot them before they spread.

We want the flowers to remain, and we want to grow new flowers in place of the weeds.

So the first lie "you aren't good enough" is one you picked up from things people have said or done to you. You've believed it because it *felt* true. We have a tendency to use our feelings to gather evidence, but feelings can and often do lie! The way you *feel* isn't actually what makes something true! Truth just *exists*! You can't *decide* what's true, you have to *discover* what's true. It turns out the truth is this: you are worthy of a good, fulfilling life where you can inspire and help those around you. You are worthy of greatness, but the second half of the lie "you can be anything you want to be" is a set-up for heartbreak. See, whoever came up with that was undoubtedly being an optimist and trying to encourage, but it's not reality. Even though what we want to be can give us a direction, desire is not enough.  A more accurate encouragement would be: You can be anything you will *work* to be. But effort isn't enough either; attitude and passion matter as well.

It takes a certain kind of person with a special kind of heart to work at Child Protective Services or at a hospital. It takes a certain kind of free spirit to commit their life to creating music or art. It takes a certain kind of individual who can understand machinery and mathematics to be an engineer or designer. It takes a certain kind of person who can perform in the spotlight to entertain people.

You are also a certain kind of person, with a certain set of gifts you were designed for, but you were *not* designed to just pick something out of a hat and go with it. You aren't just anybody that can fill any spot, you are intentionally *you*, and only you can fill that personalized place in this world. You are not everything, but you are very beautifully *something*.

You are worthy to fulfill that purpose inside of you, but you also must learn to recognize exactly what it is that fits who you are. From fifth grade through sophomore year of high school, I was confident that I was meant to be a basketball player. It wasn't until my junior year of high school that I realized basketball was not in my future plans. It was difficult to grasp, but the passion inside of me resonated with a path I had never known I could take. See, that's one of the amazing things about school, and participating in that chapter of my life. All those classes, all those clubs, all those sports — they were different options and fields and worlds I got to experience, which helped me figure out what I was good at and what I resonated with, be it at my desk or on the field. It was because of school that I learned to love football. You may be an artist, or a musician, or a caretaker, or an architect or something else, but checking in on the activities that move your spirit are going to give you major clues, even if they don't open you up completely to the "thing" you're meant to do someday.

You are absolutely worthy of greatness, because your success is not measured by the rest of the world. And … just be you.  Be the best, most authentic version that you can be. Walking in truth will allow you to be confident, touch hearts, and positively impact yourself and the world around you.

**Lie #2** — You Don't Deserve to be Happy … But You Can Have Anything You Want

Have you ever told yourself that you're too young or too old? That it's too hard to lose that weight or that you're too dumb to understand? Have you ever looked at other people's lives and craved what they had — things, success, reputation, confidence, but believed none of that's possible for you? Have you ever been told that your life has to be perfect or felt your life is harder than everyone else's? Have you ever looked at all the bad stuff that's happened to you and felt you deserved it?

I like to call these types of lies "dream-breakers". These are the ones that cause us to freeze up, or shut down, or go stagnant with indecision or complacency. They eat at your dreams like piranhas, and then one day you look back at all the things you lost out on because of those beliefs.

These beliefs like to stay for the long haul and eat away at you until there's nothing left. *Now* is the time to wage war on them!

That's easier with some inspiring examples. Remember Marcus Aurelius and Henry Ford? I'd encourage you to do a little research on them. Learn about the struggles and obstacles they faced, and how they perceived themselves through the chaos. Find out why these men and others like them didn't let the lies hold them back.

In my own life, I could have let my abuser's lie that I was weak and undeserving of anything good be my truth, but instead I sought out real truth. *Deserving* has nothing to do with happiness. Happiness is a choice we make, and it will only happen if we choose to love. Love ourselves, love others, love the opportunities given to us.

The other extreme that this lie entails — that "you can have anything you want" — gives many people the license to make cruel choices for their own happiness. The truth is, we share this world, and how we treat others in it will affect us and our success, and often theirs as well!

I counter these lies in my own life by lifting up others. Somehow it also helps me see myself more clearly. For starters, I encourage others when I see them working hard to better themselves. Whenever I see an out-of-shape person in the gym, I give them a thumbs-up or an encouraging smile, because they are there for themselves, just like I am. Whatever their goal, they are making an incredible effort to change their mindset and beliefs and to better themselves by working hard. They are not waiting around for someone to give them what they want. I'm doing the same thing when I'm in the gym. I'm contradicting any voice who ever said I can't or shouldn't bother. I'm working towards a long and meaningful future to the best of my ability.

Then there is the flip-side of the lie, getting whatever you want. If we are measuring ourselves by others' success or livelihood, then we aren't focusing on ourselves in a healthy way. Watching other people live their life and wanting what they have isn't going to make us happy. The expectation of "getting what you want" will not bring you happiness.

Even if you do get what you want, it may be fleeting. Happiness has to be found in other ways. Playing football brought me a lot of happiness while it lasted, but I did not allow my career-ending injury to crush my joy. I continued to live a life helping, inspiring and encouraging others, and my happiness has continued to flourish. It would have been easy to listen to the lies that tried to tell me my life was over because my career ground to a screeching halt. But I chose not to believe the lie that I should be unhappy because I didn't get what I wanted. I know my truth. I wasn't just meant for one thing and now it's over. I was meant to play football for a time, but I was also meant to write this book and encourage people. And my happiness is found in living my life and taking the journey and letting the flowers fill my garden.

**Lie #3** — You're a Nobody ... But You're the Only One that Matters

We can get bogged down in these lies, where we tell ourselves that we aren't anyone special, but yet we strive to be like the celebrities, entrepreneurs, and influencers we see on TV or online, who are living as though the world revolves around their ideas and opinions. The truth is, you *are* someone that matters, and you have something special to offer the world, but you don't live in a void where your actions and behaviors won't affect others. The balance is found in understanding that the place you hold in this world requires caring for yourself, but also caring for the people around you. What you do in this world matters. To yourself and to others, whether you realize it or not.

Have you ever been to a cemetery and looked at a headstone? Usually, you'll see a name, a date of birth and when that person passed away, maybe a picture engraved in the stone, and sometimes even a quote that reflects the person's character. Often you'll see a relationship noted, for example, "Beloved wife and mother." Every headstone has the name of somebody who lived and died. Each of them was special to someone else. Each of them made mistakes and learned valuable lessons. Some of them were full of happiness, some struggled to love their lives. They left a mark on the world, whether they fulfilled their dreams or not.

What is the most important part on those headstones? It's not the name or dates or decorative details. It's actually that tiny little line in between the date of birth and date of death. That little " – " represents everything about the life of the individual. Your little dash on your headstone is where every decision, struggle, fight, interaction, tear, failure, success, and smile will exist. My sophomore high school coach used to tell us, "Live the dash." Now, I'm telling you the same.

I've always liked the Nike slogan: "Don't believe you have to be like anybody to be somebody." Now that is a truth to live by. In a society like ours, we tend to feel a need to compete for success and reputation. Influencers on social media can't influence if they don't have followers, right? So they work hard to say and do the things that will get the most people to notice and follow and admire them. Sometimes that requires them to create a fake persona or do things that might be harmful to the mind or body. Many young people get negatively influenced everyday by people who *appear* to have something desirable to offer, but these influencers are rarely encouraging healthy individuality.  Of course, not all influencers are like this. Some have a genuine intent to help people be their best self, but the temptation for most people with a platform is to encourage reaching success in the same ways they have.

A common misconception we have is believing that an influencer is a leader. Words and meanings often change over time. At one point, the word influencer was synonymous with leader, but today, we tend to use that label in reference to the social media influencers we see all around us. A leader, however, is something much more powerful in a much less flashy way. While both a leader and an influencer are looked up to, and have the power to inspire people's behaviors, they also differ. The influencer *needs* people to exist, while a leader is a leader by nature and gifting. A leader doesn't need people, but people will naturally be drawn to them. A good leader will serve people with humility, while an influencer simply feeds off the adoration. Influence can and will fade with the fads, but leadership, if well developed, will be a life-long gift.

Will Smith has always wanted to change the world through his acting and hard work. He once stated, "Don't chase people. Be yourself, do your own thing, and work hard. The right people — the ones who really belong in your life — will come to you. And stay." I like to add: "And they'll believe in you."

We are all designed differently, and being unique is special because there is only one of you. You aren't a copy of someone else. You have your own ideas, thoughts, feelings, visions, dreams, and passions. The more you search out how to be someone else, the more you take away from yourself. The more you think you're a nobody, the more weeds you're allowing in your garden. Get rid of these lies. Look in the mirror and recognize you have something to offer. Not because other people validated you, but because your existence is validation enough.

# OVERTIME REFLECTION

- What lies have impacted your self-love, and how?

- What truths have people told you when you were hard on yourself?

- How do you feel when someone else sees the greatness inside of you?

# 36

# WHEN LIFE PUTS YOU IN CHECK

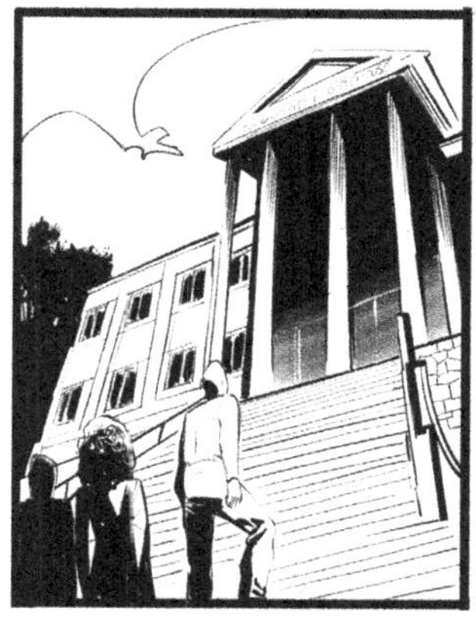

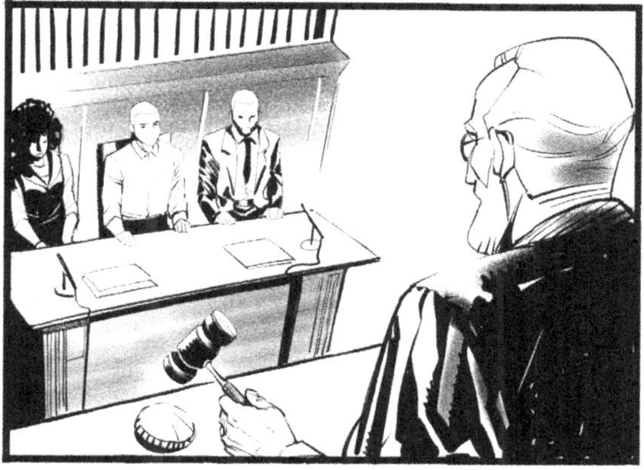

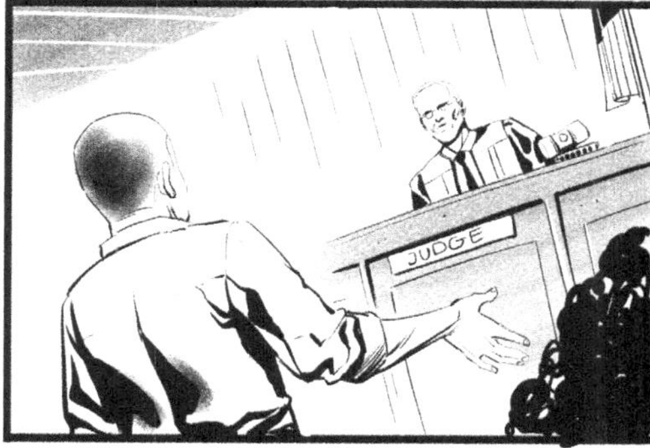


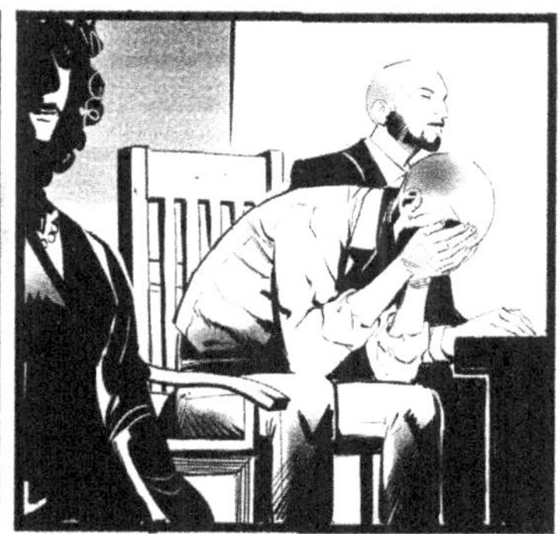

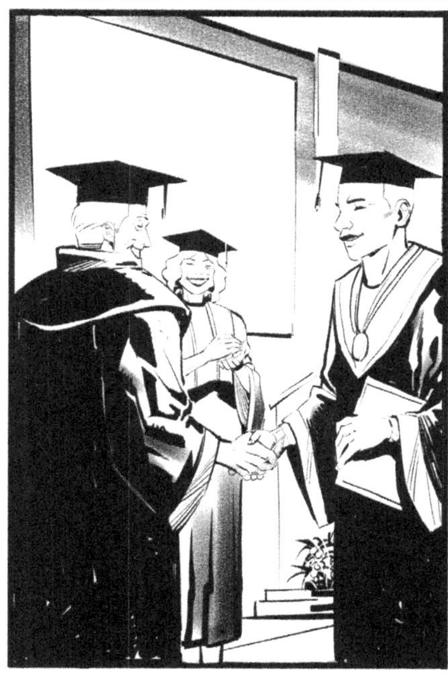

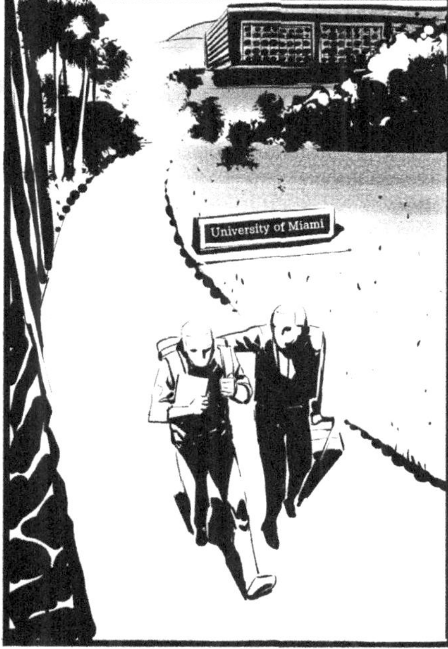


234

It was only a couple weeks after signing with University of Miami that my father, my stepmother, and I were heading to court. My abuser was trying to clear her record of the abuse in order to obtain a specific job. Having an abuse report and a past history of Child Protective Services involvement on her file wasn't looking good for her, so we were called into court to address the abuse that had happened to me seven years earlier. Somehow the fact that I was being required to testify made me feel like a pawn in a game of chess. I had no desire to be set up to look like her enemy, and even less desire to help her success.

To be honest, there were more conflicted emotions and anxiety in this single day than any day I could remember before. In the back of my mind I was terrified this court mess would impact my future. Worst of all, I had to face my abuser once again, someone I hadn't seen since middle school, and this time, she was going to hear my side of the story.

I suddenly felt like the eleven-year-old version of myself. The one who was still facing the threat of abuse on a daily basis. That traumatized little boy was still alive inside of me. I had grown into a young man by this point, but deep down inside my heart, that little boy was there, trembling in fear. He didn't want to be stepping into the courtroom any more than I did.

We arrived at the hearing, and I was surprised to see people I recognized already there; people I had once been close to. I hadn't expected to see any of their faces, and it was clear from their expressions, they weren't happy to see me. I kept my eyes forward and quietly walked past them all to my seat, my father and stepmother at my side the whole way. I wanted to be done with this ordeal as quickly as possible so I could go back to the good life I had been working so hard to build.

I was thrown off by the addition of all these onlookers. The morning of the 'incident,' there had been only two people present, Her and myself. Everyone else in this courtroom had no clue what had gone on. Not a single one had ever spoken to me about it. It was clear they were here for Her. I didn't really know what I was going to say or how I was going to respond once it was my turn to give my testimony. I felt as though I was on trial myself, which was strange because I was the victim all those years ago.

Before I was questioned by the lawyers, the judge asked my father to leave the courtroom. This was very upsetting to me, because without him I only had my stepmother in my corner. Perhaps removing my father would keep me from replicating his testimony or seeking nonverbal guidance. I'm not sure if this was the reason but it didn't matter. All I remember is the intense wave of anxiety I felt as he walked further and further away, until the doors closed behind him. It suddenly became really hard to think; my mind felt blurry.

When I took the stand, I felt exposed; naked and vulnerable. All eyes were on me. I just wanted to get through this as quickly as possible and get off the stand. The lawyers questioned me, and I gave my testimony. No more, no less.

They asked me about my abuse, asking me to rate the severity on a scale from one to ten. I told them a flat ten, but I didn't elaborate. When I sat back down, I barely remembered what I had said. My stepmother told me that my answers were very short, that I gave very little detail, and I made statements like, "I just want to live with my dad."

I listened to all the other testimonies that were in support of my abuser. When it was Her turn to take the stand, she blatantly lied. It was no surprise to me, and yet it hurt to hear her tell those lies. I bit my tongue to keep from responding and just waited.

As the court day ended, a new wave of emotion hit me, relief. I could now get back to my normal life and focus on finishing the school year strong. I had done what was required of me, and now I was moving on.

I learned later down the road that my testimony was classified as an "uncredible witness." Perhaps some people couldn't believe a seventeen-year-old, 235-pound, college-signed football player that came across as uncertain and timid. That behavior in itself should have been evidence that something was wrong, but really, it didn't matter. I hadn't gone to court to get revenge on my abuser (although she did not get the job). That wasn't my character or the man I was working to become. I didn't care what she was choosing to do with her life, I was choosing to stay focused on what I was going to do with mine.

I finished my senior year the way I needed to. I ended my high school career on a high note, and it felt good. I was looking forward to the summer because the University of Miami was the next quest of my life ... which was over 3,000 miles away from home.

# 37

## KEEP PRESSING FORWARD

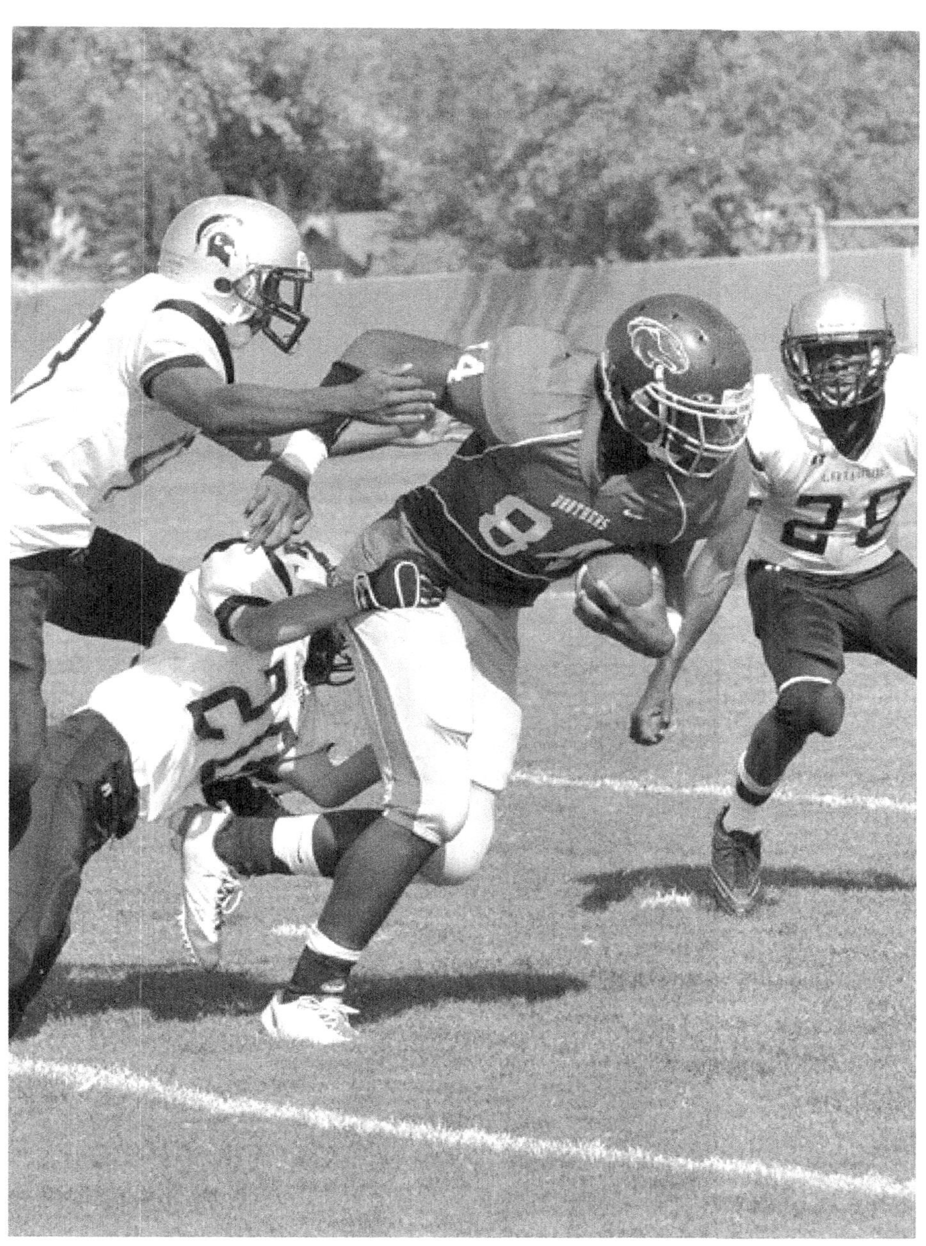

n my experience, when momentum is built up and life is moving along at a swift pace, obstacles will come along and try to stop you or slow you down. Sometimes these snags will be minor inconveniences, while others might require a detour to go around. Occasionally, you'll come up against an entire log jam attempting to bar your path and you may have no choice but to simply bust through. The court case was like that for me. There was no way I could avoid it — no way around it, over it, or under it. I had to go straight through.

While there may have been better or more effective ways for me to handle what I did or didn't address that day, it doesn't matter now. I did the best I could in the moment, and when it was all said and done, I was through the other side and continuing forward.

In your own life, I encourage you to be mindful of your surroundings, so you can recognize snags that may try to keep you from moving forward. They could come in all sorts of different forms like: an unhealthy relationship, spending too much time enjoying the pleasures of life instead of pursuing your future, struggling grades in school, poor money management, addiction, struggling to manage time wisely, internalizing negative thoughts and feelings, avoiding hard conversations, and the list goes on. Why are these snags important to recognize and overcome? Great question

As we've talked about already, success is built through struggle, but remaining in the struggle is like leaving all those weeds in your beautiful garden. It's like leaving sails up while your ship is in the middle of a hurricane. Snags, if not dealt with, can come back to haunt your life later. Some snags can be short lived while others could rip a hole in your boat that causes you to end up stalling your progress indefinitely. Either way, they can hinder us for the short or long-term. It's our job to confront the challenge and get through it the right way, but also come out the other end learning something from it.

When you are on your quest to self-discovery, you must be consciously aware of the barriers and obstacles in front of you. This allows you to be creative and flexible as you navigate. If you were to run through an obstacle course, you'd notice that some of the hurdles aren't very difficult to maneuver, but as you progress further and further through the course, the barriers and challenges would become increasingly more difficult. Some are insurmountable unless you accept help or offer help to others. Some of them take more time to get over before moving on to the next challenge. Life is most definitely an obstacle course filled with various challenges to overcome, both within yourself, and at times with the help of others.

So here is how I see the Obstacle Course of Life, you can either remain at the starting line and never move past it (fear), you can avoid the whole thing (doubt), you can give up early (failure), or … you get bruised, dirty, sweaty, exhausted, and experience excruciating pain, discover new skills you didn't know you had, and use parts of your mind and body you may not have utilized before, in order to reach the finish line. Guess which option betters you and ends with success.

Are you a big reader or movie fan? What is something we see the protagonist (hero) go through in each story? Struggles. Obstacles. Circumstances. Snags. Why? Because without them, they are flat and spiritless. These difficulties are what help us relate to these detailed characters. We resonate with their struggles and stories. We understand the hardships they face, and we go on that journey with them hoping for their best all the way to the end. We're passengers on their journey, but we're also obsessed with seeing if they overcome it all just for: a climactic ending of success, a sad ending, a happily ever after ending, a riding off into the sunset ending, an avenging ending, a hug-your-enemy ending, or a jumping-high-five freeze frame.

Here's another way of understanding our connection with storylines and conflicted characters. Have you noticed how big video games continue to get? The storylines of these characters are incredibly powerful. Yet, we have such a loyal commitment to get these characters through the storyline by any means necessary. We don't want to fail that character, because we feel the resounding disappointment each time we aren't able to get through the barriers. We are on this journey of self-discovery with the main character. We want them to succeed, and throughout the game we are earning achievements for all we've accomplished along the way.

There are so many incredible stories out in the world, and your story is one of them. What are your challenges and barriers? What achievements have you earned so far in life? What lessons have you experienced? How have these experiences shaped you?

Even though it sounds frightening to hear, failure and snags and struggle are common and necessary factors in life. We can either overcome them or avoid them entirely. Hiding from or discarding the Obstacle Course of Life hinders our individualized existence. Without the quest and struggle, we become flat and characterless ourselves. We become the "extra" in the scene, offering little to nothing to the main characters. But you aren't just another body taking up space, this is *your* story, so make your struggles and choices matter to your success! I know some of us have greater obstacles than others, but hardship is par for the course when it comes to living and surviving, like it or not.

My abuse from the age of six to the age of eleven was something I couldn't control. The court hearing at the age of seventeen was another circumstance I wasn't able to control. They were snags that tried to hold me up, but eventually I got free of them and kept moving. As we get into the next few chapters, however, you're going to see that there were some snags I did not choose to navigate wisely; barriers I put there myself that I shouldn't have allowed. You're going to see that I made mistakes because I wasn't yet consciously aware of the weeds growing in my garden. Learn from my mistakes, because some of these choices could have been detrimental to my future.

# OVERTIME REFLECTION

- When was the last time you bounced back from a tough situation?

- Has a life circumstance ever convinced you to give up?

- What methods can you use to unsnag yourself in a current situation?

# 38

# THE CATCH

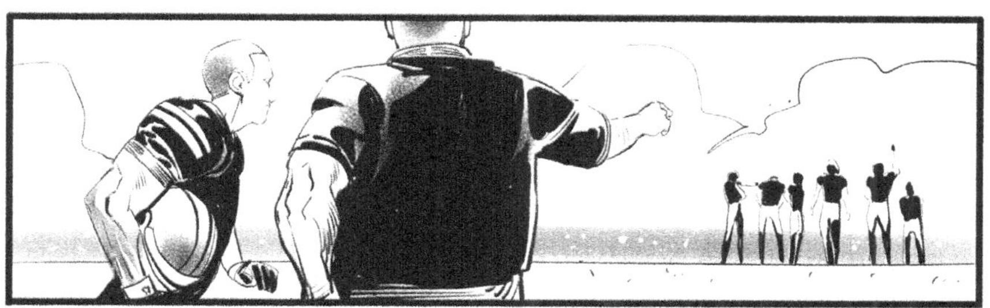

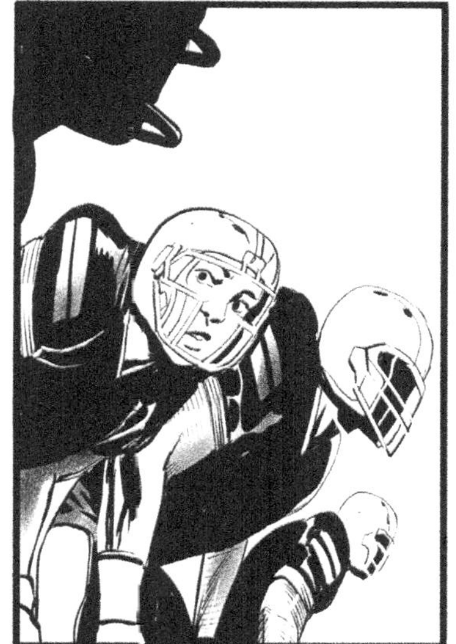

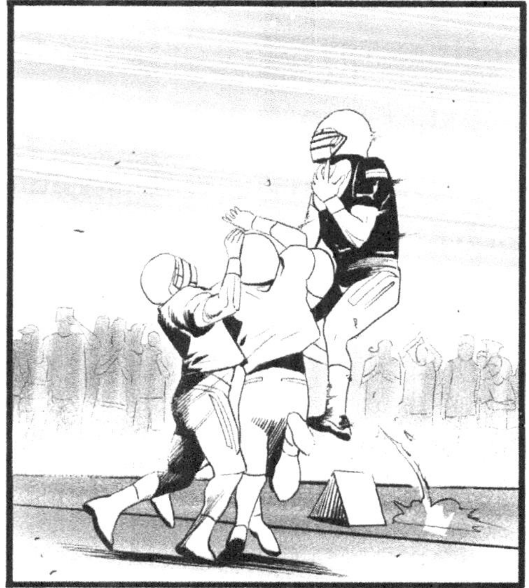

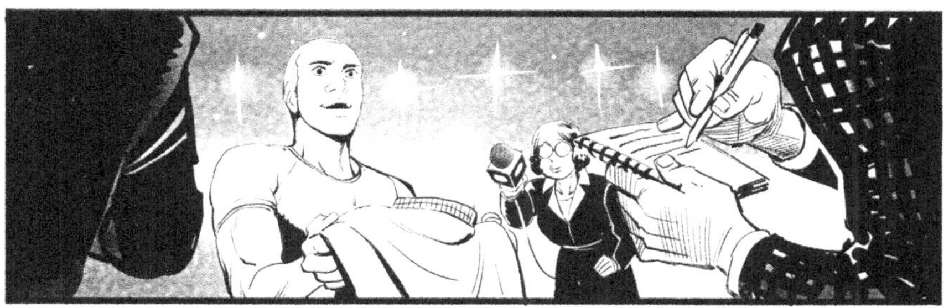

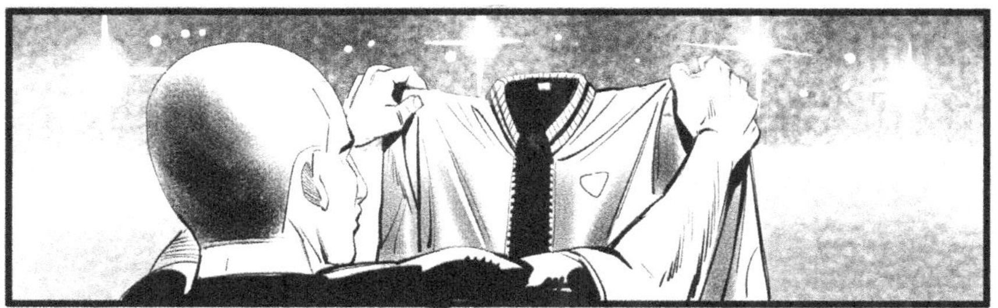

**"**No matter what school you choose, we're always a plane flight away." The voices of my dad and my stepmom kept replaying over in my head as Dad and I traversed the thousands of miles to my new college. We had left my home in Sacramento to take the trip to Miami together. My dad wanted to be there for my first week of football camp. I think me going to this high-level school was just as nerve-wracking for him as it was me. But it felt good having him around. I really cherished these father-son moments. And he was there with me every step of the way, like my guiding star. He had always been one to help me talk through stressful decisions, whether it was debating quitting football in high school, or wondering which college to attend. He had a way of playing devil's advocate that helped me look at all angles of the situation. Now he was there helping me make plans about going professional after college. Whenever I was in a bind on which direction I needed to go, he was there. He was more than my dad, he was my rock.

The transition from a private high school to a private college was drastic. The speed and pace at Miami was faster, and the culture of the school was also quite different. I had just graduated high school and already had so many things to adjust to at once. I was taking two summer college courses while maintaining the strength & conditioning regimen of the football program. This training was leaps and bounds harder compared to high school, but my agility and jump capabilities had much improved. However, the skills required to play and participate at this level of talent really made me second guess if this was what I wanted. I knew the struggle and challenge was going to make me better, but it was hard on my ego to feel so overwhelmed with these workouts. Was this the right choice, or had I made a mistake coming here?

I was 6'5" by college, but I went from being the biggest guy on the block back in high school to being just average height at the University of Miami, and even worse, all my new teammates were bigger, stronger, and faster than me. I was no longer *the big man on campus* like I once was in high school, and it really put my pride in check. I had to be resilient in my mindset, and I had to discipline myself, because two weeks later football camp started.

I was thankful my dad was able to be there for camp. He wanted to see me practice with all the other guys. He wanted to see what I had learned over the summer that led up to this point. At the start of camp, I was very hesitant in my capabilities. I had been confident a year ago, but now I wasn't so sure. The football program had recruited three other tight ends, one being the #1 JUCO tight end in the nation. (Three of us eventually went on to play in the NFL, which gives you an idea how intense the competition was for my position, even as a freshman.) But my dad had faith in me. He knew that once I walked onto the practice field for camp, I was going to do great things. And he was right.

Nervous as I was, I was ready to go. The first couple days of camp we just wore helmets, but then the crashing and smashing came soon after when we strapped on full pads, and when the pads came out the fans came out. They began flooding into the stadium early to see how their team was looking. The journalists and photographers also made appearances.

Then, an opportunity came a-knockin' one day, a chance that helped me gain attention, and I answered. During camp, there was one play that put me on both the coach's and media's radar. During a scrimmage with the defense, I ran a route. The quarterback had thrown the ball in my direction, but it was a bit high. I turned and jumped, making this incredible catch over three other defenders. To me, I was just doing my job and making the catch, but to the fans it was more. The media swarmed me after practice, and my mindset changed. I felt that I could do this.

After camp, I had achieved something amazing. I worked hard, practiced harder, and continued to demonstrate my talent. I must have done something right, because the coaches gave me a special jacket indicating I was now officially on the traveling team as a freshman. This jacket was like armor for me, it confirmed that I was one of the guys going to other stadiums to play football. I was hooked now, and as an eighteen-year-old, I would be playing with the big boys.

The first time I wore the jacket and traveled with the team was to Ohio State University, over 100,000 people filled the stadium. Let me tell you, there is a difference between being in the stands compared to being on the field. Looking up into the bleachers, I felt very small in a moment that felt larger than life. This was more than what I dreamed football would be. Just four years earlier I'd been unsure if I wanted to stick it out with football anymore, but now ... wow!

I didn't get to play half the season because I was 3rd in the line-up for my position. There was a senior tight end, the #1 JUCO tight end, and myself, but it didn't matter. I was a traveling freshman playing for the University of Miami, standing on the sidelines with my team on the field for every game. I thought it couldn't get better than this.

But I was wrong. Another amazing opportunity came when the coach put me in after halftime against Duke. Tight ends are play-makers, because when the time comes, the team depends on a tight end making the big catch or big block when necessary. And that's exactly what happened in this game. Back-to-back, I was able to make two plays that got us a first down.

On the first conversion, I made a route to the middle of the field. Subconsciously and out of habit, my eyes saw the ball and my hands raised up. I caught it and fell to the ground, and my first thought was "Oh, damn! That was cool!" Then I did it again the very next play.

I had no idea those two plays had caught the attention of the local paper until my math professor congratulated me on my performance he had read about.  Sure enough, when I got my hands on a copy, I was right there on the front page of the sports section! This was becoming real.

This put me in a whole different, more intense mindset. Each time an opportunity came calling during practice or games, I intentionally stepped up and performed exactly how I needed to. After spending all those hours and months and years on my craft, I was ready for these moments. The more prepared I became, the more I fell in love with the sport and everything that came with it.

Then, unexpectedly, I got a nasty concussion. It was early in a game against Maryland. I got tripped on a run play, and the last thing I remember was a big lineman falling on top of me. Suddenly, I was sitting on the sideline talking with a teammate and having *zero* recollection of how I got there. It also dawned on me that I wasn't really sure who we were playing. The thought came to me that we were playing Cordova, one of my high school rivals, which didn't make sense because I was pretty sure I was in college now.

The kickoff team was called by one of the coaches, so I hopped up with my helmet in hand. Jimmy, my teammate, grabbed me and sat me back down. "No way, man." He knew I was concussed, and he got me to sit out the rest of the half.

At halftime, I was heading to the locker room with the rest of the team when Coach Pannunzio came alongside me. "Asante, hey. How're you feeling?"

"I'm good, Coach. Ready to go for the second half."

He nodded and studied my eyes. "That's good to hear. I have a question for ya."

"Sure, Coach. What's up?"

"What day is it today?"

What kind of question was that? It sounds easy to answer. My first impulse was to say January, but I knew that was wrong. I just smiled at him and said, "It's game day, Coach."

Slowly and calmly, he took my helmet and told me I was done for the rest of the game. This was hard for me to accept, but I didn't fight it.

I want to give all you athletes some advice. Your

coaches (and teachers) are supposed to look out for you. To them, you are their responsibility, no matter how you feel about it. They want what is best for you. Their role is to take care of you. Please, let them, and understand where they come from.

The rest of the following week I sat out of everything — practice, gym workouts, and even the following game. The team traveled to Georgia Tech that next game, too, which really disappointed me because I had family out there. It was hard to tell everyone I wasn't going to be playing. It would have been good to see them. Instead, I watched my team play on TV from my dorm.

Two days later, a Monday, I was eating lunch in the cafeteria when a teammate came up to me. "Man, that's messed up that you didn't tell your mom that you weren't traveling this week."

My first thought was if I accidently forgot to tell my parents that I wasn't traveling to Georgia Tech, but I was pretty sure I had. They saw me get the concussion against Maryland, and they were at the doctor's appointment when I was told I had, in fact, a concussion. I looked at him perplexed. "My mom knew I wasn't playing this week. What are you talking about, man?"

He shrugged. "Well, there was a lady in the stands saying she was your mom and she was asking where you were."

Oh, damn. My caretaker and abuser didn't know I was injured, but had made a surprise visit to one of my games. That didn't make sense. She wouldn't even drive a few miles to watch one of my high school games, so why all of a sudden would she fly across the country for a college game? And then it hit me. She had family in Georgia, which was probably her excuse to fly thousands of miles for the game.

Sighing and collecting my thoughts, I explained to my teammate my relationship with Her. He understood quickly. Shifting the conversation back to the game, I tried to play it cool and move on. But on my way to class, I called my dad and told him.

He chuckled, and then added, "Well, everything happens for a reason."

How right he was. The one game She showed up to was the game I wasn't allowed to play. Obviously, I wasn't supposed to be at that game. Even when something happens that seems negative, just consider the possibility that there is a bigger reason for it.

The first game back after the doctor cleared me from my concussion, I was the starting tight end against Virginia Tech. We lost the game. We then lost the following game against South Florida University, which placed us in the

Sun Bowl against Notre Dame, which we also lost. It had been a miserably cold game too, and we knew it was going to be a losing game for us the moment we walked onto the field. All of us were wearing long sleeves, hand-warmer pouches, and heat-insulated visors. Our opponents wore short sleeve shirts. They were used to the cold, we were not. It played a huge factor in our loss.

Despite the losses, I was really happy with how my first college football season went. I had also done well in my academics, maintaining a 3.3 grade point average and making the academic honor roll. But with all the attention I gained from football, my ego started to inflate. I demonstrated poor judgments in my character and began to feed off all the attention from fans and peers. I was loving the spotlight. Being 'The Guy' on the team was a lot for an eighteen-year-old to handle, and I definitely didn't handle it well. I started to become more and more distracted by these things going into my sophomore year.

After the bowl game, though, my position coach, Coach Pannunzio, noticed me having problems with my shoulder, so he directed me to the athletic trainer. After some scans and tests, they discovered that I had torn my labrum, requiring surgery. The procedure meant I was pulled from playing as I continued to heal and do physical therapy. Meanwhile, winter training was going on.

Around this time, we also got a new coaching staff. As the new guys were doing their assessments and evaluations of all the athletes, I was still healing and I couldn't be there to demonstrate my strength and skills. My reputation of being 'The Guy' dropped, and I was no longer the top dog tight end. Because of this uncontrollable circumstance, I dropped in the depth chart, coming into camp weaker. I had lost so much time working on my craft and building my body, but I couldn't force the healing process, otherwise the natural consequence would have been reinjury.

During this time in my sophomore year, because my pride was no longer being fed, I caught myself on a snag. My attitude turned sour and bitter. I became selfish in my perspective that year. I blamed others for my loss of progress, and instead of getting focused I got distracted. One day in a meeting, the coach caught me falling asleep. He ripped into me, loudly calling me out for my lack of respect. In practice directly after that, I messed up on 3 different plays. And just like that, I was off the traveling team within 24 hours. It had taken years to get where I was, and just a few moments of carelessness and distraction to lose it. My high school sophomore football coach, Coach Lahey, said it best: "One 'oh shit' can wipe out a thousand 'attaboys.'" I now knew what he meant.

Football was not okay for me that year. We had

finished with six wins and six losses, but we served a self-imposed bowl ban due to an ongoing NCAA investigation that was discovered in 2010. A scandal was uncovered, and it was something that had gone on in the athletics department behind closed doors for over a decade. Due to the probing, we dropped out of the bowl game. The snags, both the ones of my own doing as well as the ones out of my control, began springing up all around me, and by my junior year, my journey was starting to take a hard turn.

# 39

# PREPARE FOR OPPORTUNITIES

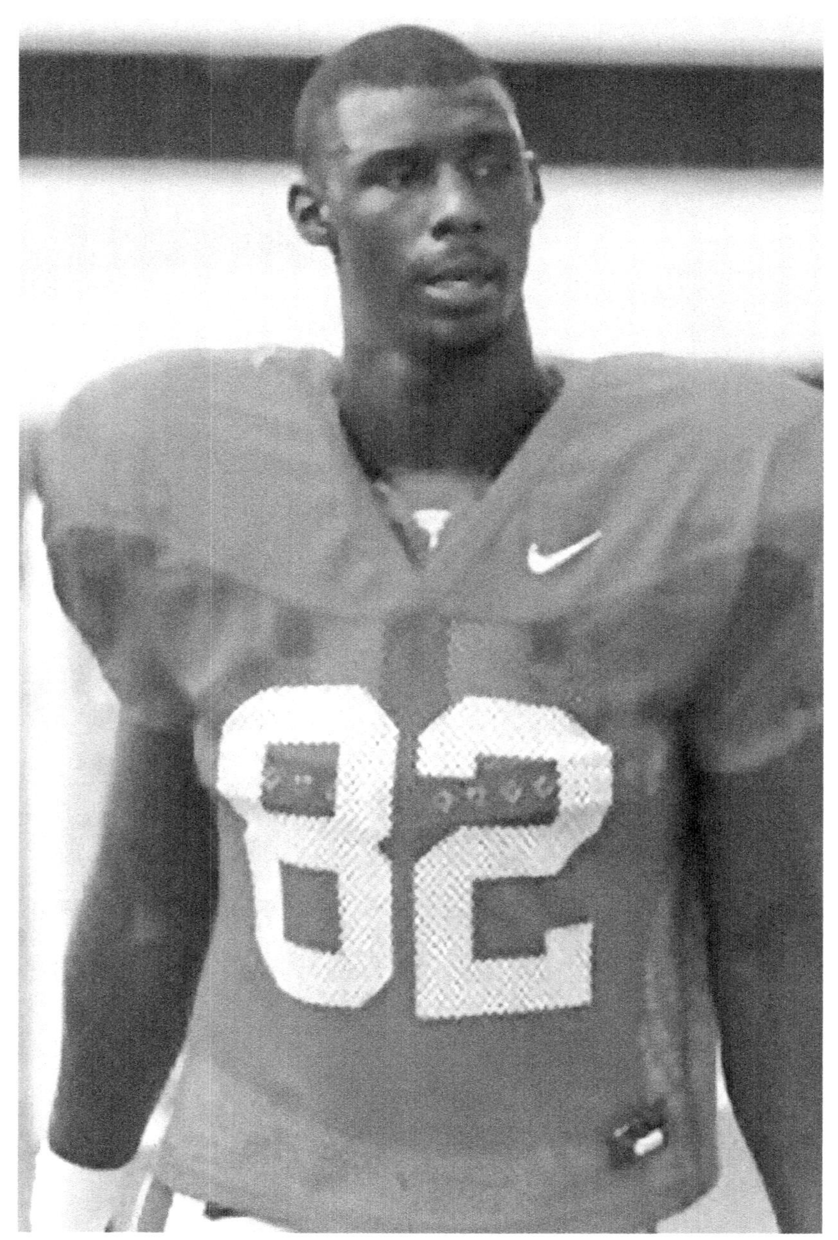

Denzel Washington once had something to say about opportunity: "I say luck is when an opportunity comes along and you're prepared for it." Opportunities are a unique thing because they never come around the same way twice. They're always different, popping their mysterious faces up randomly and spontaneously throughout our lives. And when we aren't aware of the direction we're taking in life, we don't really know how to recognize the opportunities that cross our path.

If I had chosen the path of playing basketball in college, none of these football opportunities would have existed because my path would have gone a different direction. I wouldn't have worn that special jacket for the traveling team. I wouldn't have made that big catch at football camp that put me in the spotlight. I wouldn't have started against Virginia Tech as a freshman. Had I chosen to stick with Washington State University instead of going to Miami, again I would've been on an entirely different path with different opportunities and outcomes as well.

So, how do you recognize opportunities that come along your path? Look at it this way: have you ever bought a car, and then suddenly start to notice how many *other* people are driving that very *same* type of vehicle? You never really pay too much attention to what people actually drive unless you have one yourself, right? Well, that same idea applies to noticing an opportunity when you take a certain path. Once something starts to matter to you, you start to see the opportunities that come with it. My path became clear when the scholarships came my way for football — not basketball. I noticed the athletic and academic opportunities that were available in Miami. I took on the challenge to take the football program's strength and conditioning training seriously. I worked my butt off during the summer. Every day I worked hard at practice because every day at practice was an opportunity, and I had to be my best. I needed to showcase my craft. The harder I worked, the more opportunities started popping up. Had I not worked hard for what I wanted, I would've missed out on so much.

And trust me when I say that it takes time to build your craft, but over that span of time, more and more opportunities make appearances. If you're prepared, then you can jump on whatever those opportunities have to offer. Thomas A. Edison was quoted, "Opportunity is missed by most people because it comes dressed in overalls and looks like work."

Now, there's another part to all this that we'll get into later, but I want to add that my journey wasn't full of sunshine and rainbows, not every day was enjoyable and fun and motivating and successful. I struggled quite a bit, mentally and physically. My body always hurt, my head hurt, my muscles hurt, I didn't sleep a lot, I couldn't visit family much, and I couldn't take days off from school. There were days I didn't want to do conditioning or hit the gym. There were days when I didn't want to be a football player. There were days I wanted to rest and relax ... but I had to remember two things: (1) I had a dream and (2) I was competing for that dream. Put yourself in my shoes: would you have given in to those excuses, knowing the outcome was possible failure? Would you have quit or taken a break, knowing it could lead you off your path? Or would you have done everything it took for those opportunities to keep flooding in?

What I want you to understand is that those hard things are part of the journey. They aren't necessarily some indication that you are on the wrong path, or that you're failing, or anything like that. They are natural by-products of working extremely hard, and still having a lot of mental, emotional, and physical barriers to work through. When life gets hard, just work through the 'suck.' Don't be anxious if you struggle, it's a sign you are still moving forward. Success is built from struggle. Seeds have to grow through the dirt of life to become a tree. If you work hard to build your skills and your craft, you'll notice these opportunities more. Time has a special way of opening doors at the right moments, and I want you to be ready for them. Work on mastering your skills, and then passion starts to grow.

If you're expecting instant success and a speedy climb to an executive role right after graduation, then you'll most likely experience quite a bit of disappointment. We can't expect the best, if we don't give our best. It won't be handed to you, you work for it. Look at Olympic athletes — these men and women are known as 'the best of the best of the best.' They invest thousands of hours to build their craft just for a few moments of glory. They are patient, resilient, and disciplined. They know what's on the line, so they have to be hyper-focused on their goals.

If you are working at your craft (writing, singing, dancing, painting, public speaking, carpentry, sports, debate, programming, architecture, farming, coding, inventing, anything really), then there will be more chances to showcase your talent and achieve whatever opportunities your future holds, because you'll be ready for them. But if you aren't preparing for these opportunities, you'll miss them. You can't be sleeping in every day or staying up late watching TV. You can't make it a habit to space out on social media or play long hours on your video games. Don't waste your time and money drinking all night with friends, because you'll waste even more time recovering the next day. Many times, disappointment will hit us hard because we fall short on an opportunity, which leads us to giving up early or moving on to something else. What's worse, we may resist taking accountability for our failure or mistake, so we handle the outcome poorly.

So, how do we prevent laziness and procrastination? First, recognize the difference between motivation and discipline. Motivation means feeling an *urge* to work, while discipline is doing the work in spite of your feelings. If you're waiting for motivation to hit you, then you're already falling behind. If you are disciplined, setting that alarm clock, sticking to a productive routine, pushing yourself just a little further than last time, then you're building momentum in the right cirection. If you have a goal, then don't waste time. Start now. Plant those seeds.

All too often people sit and wait for an opportunity to come to them, or hope life is going to magically pick a path for them. But, if you don't know what path you want to take, then how are you going to know what an opportunity looks like when it shows up? Great question. We probably won't see the opportunity because we don't know what we're looking for, because we're not choosing a direction to go. You're placing yourself in limbo, by choice. Remember what I said earlier — take the first step, then the second step, and then follow through. Be patient and build your craft. If you take the first step and then sit down, then how do you expect to get anywhere? You won't, and you'll have no one to blame but yourself.

Maybe some of you have been working for years towards something and nothing seems to be happening yet. Is it too late for you? Let me give you a few examples of people who built their craft *while* waiting for their opportunity to pop up. Colonel Sanders didn't get his big break for KFC until his sixties. Nelson Mandela became president of his country at 76 years old *after* serving 27 years in jail. Samuel L. Jackson spent decades in small bit roles until he was 43 years old, which was when he finally landed his first time role in the award-winning Spike Lee film, *Jungle Fever.* Julia Child was fifty years old when she wrote her first cookbook that launched her career. Laura Ingalls Wilder started writing in her later years in life, publishing her first books after the age of sixty. Her stories became literary classics and the basis for the hit TV show, *Little House on the Prairie.*

These individuals are shining examples of what discipline and resilience looks like. They spent years and decades building their craft. When opportunities finally came, they were prepared and ready. If they had sat in their bedrooms doing nothing, the world would never have known their names, or benefited from what they had to offer. This is how we should all see our futures. You may be a president, or an author, or just the creator of really good chicken, but no matter which path or skill you've been given, it's something that only *you* have to offer. Every path is different, and no opportunity comes with a manual, but nothing can ever be achieved without effort. And sometimes you succeed without getting any acclamation for many years.

In our instant gratification society, we are seeing bad habits in job-hopping and an increase in workers who are unhappy with their job. Do an experiment: ask parents, guardians, grandparents, aunts, uncles, teachers, cashiers, secretaries, principals, or your boss if they're doing their dream job? Some will say yes, some will say no, and some will say they grew into it. Our culture right now is less inclined to work towards something. We are so used to having our packages arrive the next day, our apps downloaded in seconds, and all the information we can dream of at our fingertips the moment we wonder about it. So working for years towards a goal isn't something a lot of people are inclined towards anymore. Patience and persistence are becoming lost arts.

There are many reasons people may not achieve the job they dreamed of as a child. Sometimes dreams have to be put on hold due to unexpected life circumstances. Sometimes people stop loving the path they thought they wanted and instead move on to another, until they land something with good pay, benefits, and a retirement plan. And that's fine, there's nothing wrong with landing a great job with good pay and benefits. Sometimes the priority is simply to put food on the table and clothes on our kids' backs. I get it, responsibility is vital, but don't give up on your craft. Spend time building your skills towards your dreams — ten minutes reading, twenty minutes researching, thirty minutes practicing, however much you can get. Don't give up that dream that was put inside of you. You may need to simply work an uninteresting job for a time, but if you never give up working on yourself and your craft, there may come a day where the door of opportunity for you to do your *thing* opens up, and you'll be ready!

What I want you to take out of this chapter is that the more you work on your skills the better you will be at it. The better you are at your craft, the more opportunities you'll see pop up on your path. Will you be ready for it? Will you take that chance and go after it? Will you be patient even when your path seems too unfulfilling and too empty?

Those are the right questions.

# OVERTIME REFLECTION

- When was the last time you took advantage of an opportunity? How did that impact you?

- What are you doing to prepare yourself for the next opportunity?

- How long are you willing to wait for that next door to open?

# 40

# GETTING IN MY OWN WAY

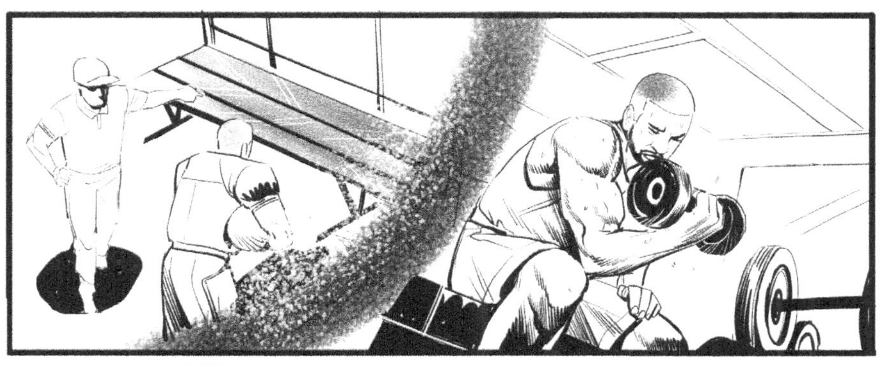
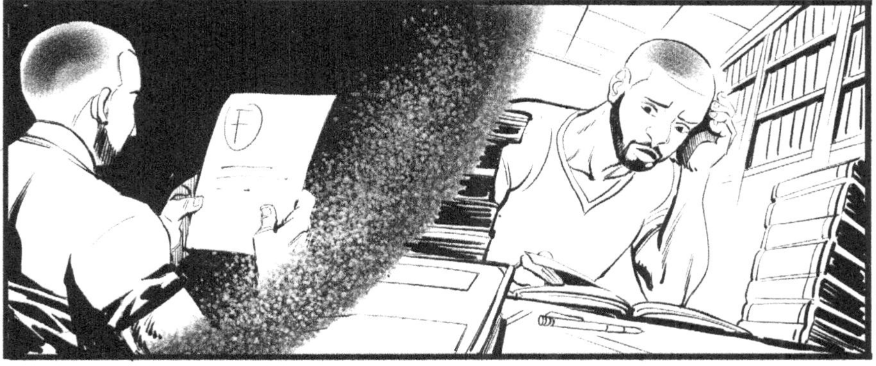
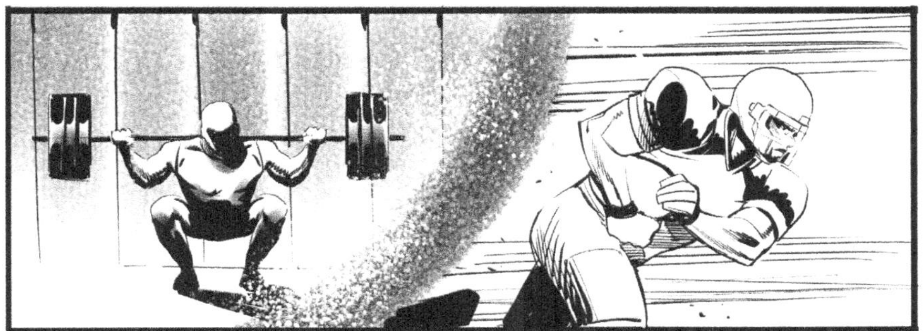
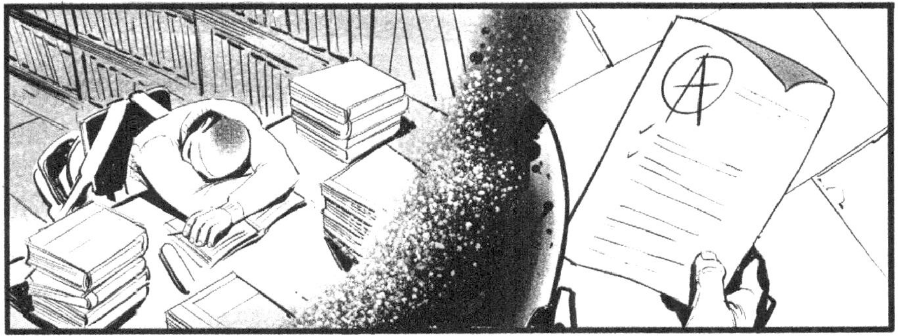

The winter after my sophomore season, the team had an entire month off due to the dropped bowl game, so I went home to my parents. Rather than sit around in my frustrations, I chose to get back on the horse and get myself into shape. Being taken off the travel team had been extremely upsetting for me, and my attitude had been partly to blame. My dad had said something at that time that helped me change my negative mindset. He said, "You have your head in the lion's mouth. The first thing you do is *don't* move and make things worse. Next, you pet the lion." He, of course, was talking about the new coaching staff. "You need to make it work between you and the coaches. You need to do what they say and work better with them." But then he added something, a bit of perspective.

When I was taken off the travel team, I had been placed on the scout team at practice. That meant that during practices, I was mimicking our opposing team's offense plays against our 1st team defense. My dad was able to point out to me that every day I would be practicing against top level defense. This would improve my craft and help me bounce back. He was giving me wisdom to see the opportunity that I hadn't noticed.

So in the meantime, while I was away from my team

for an entire month, I trained hard. I spent every day in the gym, pushing myself harder than before. There were days I puked from exhaustion, but my mindset was fixed. No one — not me or the coaches or anyone else — was going to get in my way. I wanted to come back as a different person. I worked in the dark, where no one else saw me excel. I trained when others slept. I took advantage of those early and late hours.

After morning training, I headed over to my high school where my old coach, Coach Wiley, was running routes with his athletes. He let me be a part of the group. I improved my craft through practicing with high schoolers, and it was awesome. These kids worked hard because I was there, and I worked hard because they were in my corner. I felt a part of something, and it was a moment I will never forget.

When I returned to school for spring training, I passed my 225 pound bench test, exceeding the number of reps the coaches had set for me, pressing up two reps more than they expected. We then jumped right into U Tough training sessions, which lasted two to three weeks and started at 5:30am. It sucked setting a 4:31 a.m. alarm, but it had to be done. I was going to discipline my way back to the top, no matter how hard I had to work.

U Tough evaluations went by a rating scale, indicated

by specific colored jerseys. The top level of skills in the assessment was a black jersey. Below that was orange, then green, then white at the bottom. I scored all black jerseys, highest rating in the tight end position. I was staying focused on me; competing with myself and not the other guys. I had to dig *myself* out of this hole that I had put myself in. No one else could.

By the end of summer camp, I was named the starting tight end again, and it felt great to get back at the top of the depth chart. Then, some unforeseen circumstances came into play. Even though I was a junior starting in the games, I wasn't playing much. I'm not a very confrontational person, so I wasn't saying anything to the coaches about their decision to pull me out, but I was missing more and more opportunities. Then the coaches unexpectedly moved two defensive ends to the tight end position. *My* position. Converting them was fine, but then these two guys started playing more than I was! What in the hell was I doing wrong? My frustration was starting to weigh down my mind, but I tried to maintain a good attitude. I didn't want to lose focus again. Even though I was becoming unhappy, I kept myself in check.

Unfortunately this inner emotional battle was once again distracting me academically. My self-worth had dropped, as well as my self-confidence. I wasn't getting the attention I needed and wanted as a player, so I sought it out elsewhere — girls. This was a big mistake, because instead of this helping clear my head, it was creating even more unhealthy distractions. During that semester, my grade point average went from a 3.3 to a 1.8, placing me on academic probation. My balance was falling apart, and the more I scrambled to control everything, the more everything crumbled from my grasp. At the time, I never linked my thought process with football to my focus in the classroom, but they were definitely connected and feeding one another. What I didn't see was that the struggles within myself were following me on and off the field. As Confucius says, "no matter where you go, there you are."

I wasn't even halfway through the season, and I was already ready to throw in the towel and transfer to another school. I wanted to change paths and look for greener grass. I didn't feel appreciated or cared about where I was, and it put me at a new low. Against North Carolina State I dropped a pass ... a touchdown pass, which would have been my first in my college career. At this point, I was so fed up with mistake after mistake, that I couldn't handle the disappointment anymore. Towards the end of the North Carolina State game, the coach called a timeout and got the offense in a huddle. He wanted a certain play to be done that required me to block. The big blocking responsibility overwhelmed me and I panicked. In my head, I felt I was going to mess things up again, so slowly and cowardly I stepped away from the huddle and found a bench to sit on. The coaches didn't know where I was, so they found someone else to replace me … or should I say I allowed myself to be replaced. I had lost my courage. And without courage, doubt came and took its place.

My team ended up winning that game with an unbelievable Hail Mary, on the same play I was supposed to be a part of. The guy who had filled my spot came out ready to play and did his job well. He came prepared, and he dominated his responsibility. I was sick about it. We finished the season seven to five with no help from me. I was lost all over again. I felt like everything had fallen apart, and my self-destructive mindset was backing up this belief. With the self-imposed bowl ban, we had another month off at the end of the season. I went home and cried. For two weeks I wallowed in self-pity, doing nothing. I didn't want anyone to help me out of my self-imposed hole of emotional darkness. I sulked and marinated in my selfishness. Before I knew it, I was fourteen pounds over my goal weight for winter training. My lack of self-regulation and self-care was showing.

In my desire to hide away from everything, I had neglected both my body and my responsibilities. In a frantic attempt to get back on track, I cut the excess weight with a terrible crash diet consisting mostly of water. The only plus side to this method was my mental determination to meet my goal before training.

Then things started looking up. One of the coaches — one I didn't get along with — had moved to a different school, and was replaced by Coach Scott. This dude was awesome. I really liked him. In a few short weeks, he was able to help me regain faith in myself again. He believed in me, and I felt like he genuinely cared. He became a bright spot when I was in my darkest place.

One day, he said, "When wishing won't, work will," spurring me to take action. Anyone can dream up an ideal scenario, but if they don't put in the work, nothing will happen. I resonated with that, and the timing couldn't have been more perfect for me to hear those words of inspiration. So, I made another change. If I was going to take this path of football, I had to do it with my all. I could no longer self-sabotage or allow my emotions to decide my future. It was time I truly worked through my obstacles and overcame my trials of self-doubt.

My grade point average bumped up to a 2.6 before the end of my junior year, getting me off academic probation. I wrote myself the following statement, and throughout that summer, I read it to myself every single day:

IT ONLY TAKES ONE YEAR

I knew this was the year that was going to get me to the professional level. I couldn't care about glory or the spotlight or touchdowns. My goal was to become the best blocker I could be for my team. I wanted the coaches to feel desperate to have me on the field during any and all run plays or passing plays. I wanted them to feel like they couldn't go a single play without me on that field. I wanted them to depend on me.

By this point, I had the support, the mindset, the discipline, and the work ethic, but I still had to focus and avoid distractions. Many of my teammates carried that same feeling, and together we went into my senior year strong, both in the mind and body. We were a solid team with a confident coaching staff — especially Coach Scott — who really helped us see our potential. I came out of summer camp named as the starting tight end, and I was *not* going to let that be taken away from me again.

We knew our team was unique by our second game of the season. We were playing #12 ranked team, Florida. It was a beast of a game. There were nearly 77,000 people in those stands and we played on ESPN with millions of viewers watching us. Winning that game, as well as the first seven games of the season, placed us at #7 in the nation. We were unstoppable.

Then there was a sudden shift. We were playing the #3 ranked team, Florida State — who later went on to win the National Championship that year. We got smoked, losing by 27 points. This put us in a funk, which impacted us for the next two games. We weren't sure what was going on, but we came up with three losses back-to-back-to-back. These weren't even close games, they were bad losses. It was like we were suddenly a different team.

We weren't happy about the change, so we did something about it. As a team, we put our heads together, and crawled out of our hole. A unified group; we were one. We came back winning the next game against Virginia, and that lit a flame under our butts. Then, in the following game against Pittsburgh, I made my first touchdown catch. All those years of work and pain and dedication had led up to this incredible feeling! When we won that game, I was on cloud nine.

Then we played the #18 ranked team, Louisville, in the Russell Athletic Bowl — our first bowl game since I was a freshman — and got creamed. We lost by 27 points in front of over 55,000 fans while playing on ESPN. It was painful losing such a big game at the end of my college career, but aside from that, we had an incredible season and we grew together as a family.

I was at a high point in my life journey. Despite the

losses, by this chapter, my spirit was unbreakable because my mindset was unbreakable. With the season over, and half of the year left of academics, my focus was now on one thing.

The NFL.

# 41

# THE BEST LAWN

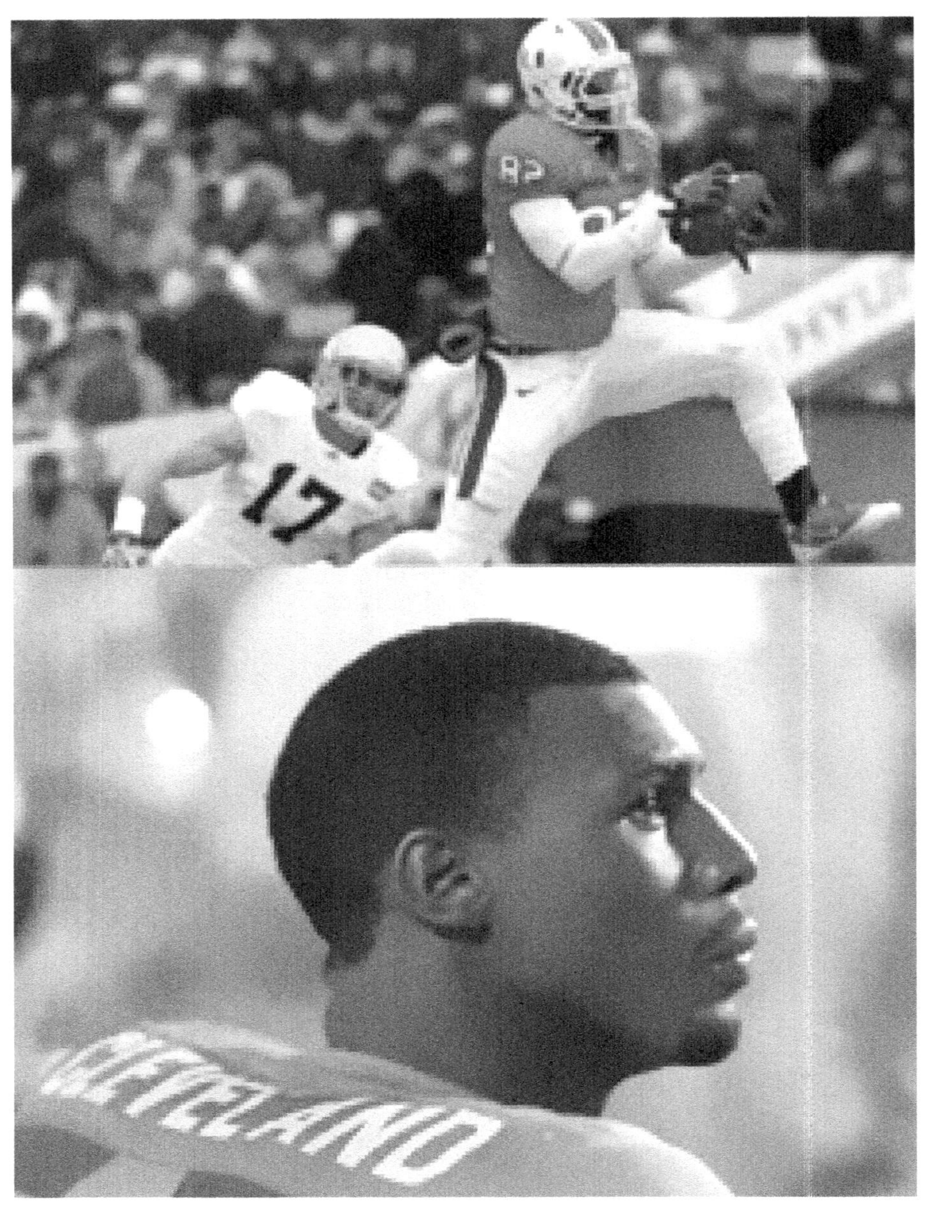

n the previous chapter, you read how uncontrolled circumstances and circumstances of my own creation nearly pushed me to quitting. You read how I nearly transferred to a new school because self-doubt had crept itself back in like a phantom. This is going to be an important thing to address in this chapter, because I want to focus on something many of us never think about as teenagers.

I'm sure you've heard the phrase, "The grass is greener on the other side," right? This sort of has a double meaning to it, but I want to take some time and explain it out for you. I want to share a perspective on this phrase that I hope helps you think a little bit more about what you already have and how to use what you already have to work towards your own greener grass.

This mindset that *the grass* on the other side of the fence *is greener*, or another way of putting it, *life is better and full of more possibilities over there*, is a trickster of a thought. This way of thinking can really damage your perspective and your own philosophy of how you see yourself, as well as how you see yourself fitting into the world around you. If we perceive the other side as being better than the side you're on, then it takes the focus off where you're at and what you already have. So what does this mindset sound like?

Have you ever made statements like: "Once I get this job, then everything will calm down," or "Once I'm done with this year, everything will be easier," or "if I just had a boyfriend/girlfriend, everything would be good," and so on and so forth? Have you ever compared your life to another person (teammate, celebrity, entrepreneur, wealthy person, captain of the team, smartest kid in school), coveting what they had, how they looked, the way they walked, the music they listened to, the car they drove, the way they talked, or clothes they wore? Did you ever think life could be so much easier having their life or getting a job like theirs or owning their things? This trickster of a mindset is a distraction tactic to keep us from being conscious of ourselves. Sure, passing daydreams are fine, but fixating on what we don't have hurts us more than helps us.

Have you ever made decisions based on the benefit or blame of another person like: choosing a college that was similar to or closest to your boyfriend or girlfriend? Did you ever make a decision to go to a college where all your friends were going or because it's where your parents pushed you to go? Did you quit piano or theatre because your teammates were picking on you? Did you ever quit Boy Scouts because you were bullied? Did you ever want to drop a class because you hated the teacher? Have you ever quit a job because you didn't get along with your boss? Did you and your friends ever target another kid because you were insecure and wanted to fit in?

"The grass is greener on the other side" is just a simple way to make excuses, to avoid being accountable for your own path. See, the truth of the matter is, grass is just grass, no matter which side of the fence it grows on. What is over there, is going to be just as complicated as what is over here, but from a distance you can't see those challenges. The grass you are in right now, is the grass you are meant to tend to if you want success. So what does this grass even represent in our lives? In order to understand this concept more myself, I had a conversation with my friend Alex, who happens to be something of an expert on lawn care.

I gave him a little bit of information about what I wanted to address in this chapter and that I wanted a little bit of feedback on what it takes to green up your own grass. Here's what he told me:

> Grass can grow just about anywhere, but to be the greener side of the grass, you need to understand how grass grows.
>
> First, be patient. Becoming the greenest yard takes a lot of patience. When I first started researching about 'how to make my lawn the greenest in the neighborhood,' I was

discouraged about how long it would take. But when you set a goal that you truly want, you'll be forced to accept being patient. You cannot expect a living thing that grows to change immediately.

You have to accept the fact that results won't happen overnight and could take years to realize.

Second, check unseen factors. While grass is the outward product that we see, it's actually the soil that is most important. I test the soil for all of the macronutrients (nitrogen, potassium, and phosphorus) and micronutrients (iron, calcium, boron, etc.). In doing this, I have an idea of what nutrients may have excessive levels and others that may be lacking. From there, I can determine the appropriate food (fertilizers) to get the soil to be a place that grass loves to grow in.

Always remember to feed your soil.

Third, get into good cultural habits. Cultural habits are the ways that we maintain the grass, keeping it healthy and growing year after year without needing to spend unnecessary hours to help it along. Letting grass grow long and cutting off more than 1/3 of it at a time stresses it and actually hurts the plant. Cutting regularly when it needs it, is vital to always having green grass. If you want to have the greenest grass, you might have to cancel other plans once in a while to take care of these basic needs.

Making consistent good habits will keep you on the right track.

Fourth, a razor sharp focus on the goal. This might be the most important part. Focusing on the long-term goal means having many little goals that keep you going on the right path. Maybe the first year, your plan is to get rid of the weeds in your yard even if the grass doesn't look great by the end of the year. Putting down herbicides (medicine) specific to each type of weed is the most effective way to reach this goal. Once you've eliminated the weeds, then the next year is adding the appropriate food to the soil. As you get the right nutrients and build better habits you will see big improvements over time.

Now you're rolling.

We had also discussed when things don't go according to

plan, to which Alex replied:

> Unfortunately, when life throws you curveballs (and it will), your goal will take a backseat because we all have responsibilities other than what we want for ourselves. THIS IS OKAY. You've already spent time building good habits and amending your soil, so if you have to neglect the yard for a little while, don't worry. It will bounce back with just a little bit of focus and a little extra patience. You'll have already learned so much more than you ever thought through your journey. You're familiar with your lawn and everything it'll take to make it great again.

All of this lawn-talk is just to say, this is the mindset you need to have in order to get where *you* want to go. If your vision of your future is dying, dead, or gone, then start putting in the work and tend to it. Don't just watch idly by as another person tends to their lawn. Don't expect others to take care of it for you. Be deliberate with your own path, choices, behaviors, and philosophy. Be curious about your future.

Alex stated that in order to have the best lawn, you need good soil. Think of it this way: feed your mind the good stuff; feed it the right stuff. Start looking for the bright spots in your life. Talk to a mentor, find a life coach, listen to motivational videos that inspire, research the craft that interests you, take personality tests and assessments, volunteer your time to a cause, ask people questions and listen, or journal your struggles, hopes, aspirations, and desires. Get rid of those toxic relationships. Turn off your phone. Catalog your progress. Be accountable for your time and choices at home and school. Be deliberate about what you put into your brain. Read books that focus on the areas/fields of work you want to be in. Read autobiographies of your role models. Set goals and work towards them. Discipline yourself and be patient because resilience is a big key factor.

What do you think would have happened to me if I had thrown in the towel when the obstacles of life got too hard? What could have happened had I transferred away? When I was at my lowest, it was not just me who got me out of the dark places. The help also came from others, people who taught me to believe in myself again. It was nutrients to my soil. It made me feel better. It helped me grow again.

I've said it a few times already, but I'm going to say it again. I believe in you. You may not believe in yourself, but at least take the first and second step towards your hopes, and then follow through. Your path may change, but you've already started the journey and gained perspective. Over time, you'll face new obstacles, and there will be times in life when your philosophy will change, as did mine. That's okay.

When barriers pop up, knock them down and learn from them. Weed out the bad and tend to your mind, body, and spirit. Don't quit. You may not realize how many people depend on you, or how many people are watching. Keep carefully and lovingly tending to the life you have right now, and you're going to end up being the best lawn in the neighborhood.

# OVERTIME REFLECTION

- What do you tell yourself to stay motivated and disciplined?

- Have you ever quit something you shouldn't have? How did it feel?

- What are you willing to change in order to achieve your dream?

# 42

# KEEP CLIMBING

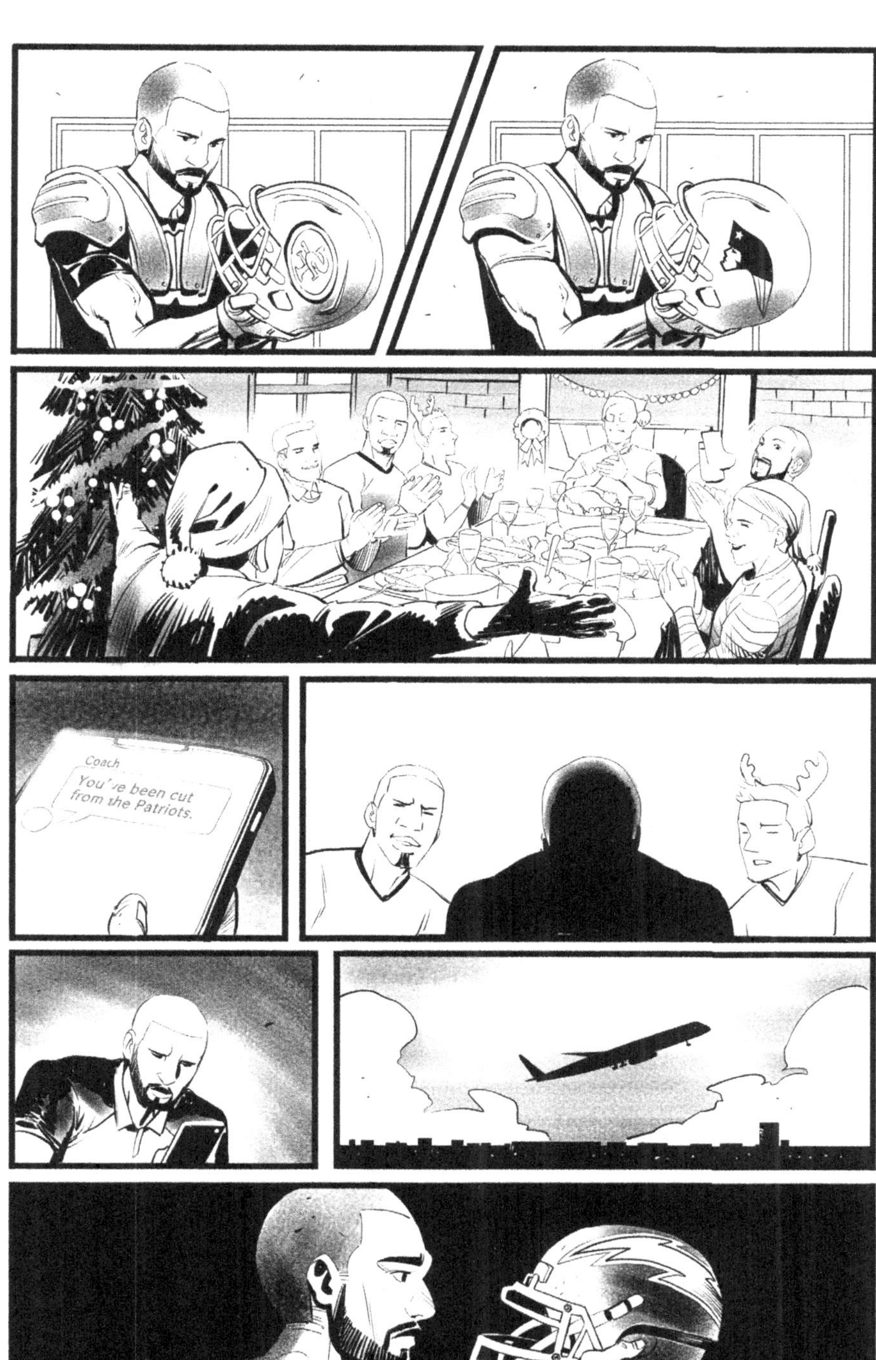


294

At the end of my senior year, I had earned the Nick Chickillo Most Improved Player Award. That award said it all. The coaches saw the work I had put in, and I never gave up on my team. After that, I got invited to play in the NFL Player Association Collegiate Game — kind of like the high school senior bowl game, but for college — where I got a touchdown.

When that was done and the season was officially over, my mind was set on one thing — Pro Day, which was in March. I wanted nothing more than to make it into the NFL. I focused on crushing all my classes, and then trained with my strength coach and a few other teammates. All of us were hyper-focused on the same thing. The competitive drive pushed us as a group. Now, the big challenge for me was that I didn't have jaw-dropping college stats. I had finished my four years at Miami with fourteen catches and 151 yards. So I knew that all of my focus would have to go to performing my best on Pro Day in front of those scouts. I had set a few goals for bench press, vertical jump, and the forty meter sprint. I knew the coaches assessed the athlete's strength, agility, and speed.

Academically, I was intensely focused. I simplified my life. I went to class, put in my training with the guys, and then went back to my dorm to complete my school work. There was no way I was going to let my education fall through my fingers. My future was certain, so my education was a backup plan in case life threw me another curveball. I had to stay focused. I didn't go out and party. I didn't allow girls and other distractions to pull me away from my goals. If I wanted down time, I watched *Breaking Bad* alone in my dorm.

During that time leading up to Pro Day, I took a couple trips around the country to visit with professional teams like the Arizona Cardinals and was even invited to meet with the Miami Dolphins. Also, a coach from the Philadelphia Eagles came to visit me. It was all just conversation though, because Pro Day was still my goal. I didn't want to rush anything like I had done back in high school. I needed to be patient and take my time.

Pro Day *finally* came and my school hosted the event. Coaches and photographers and journalists were everywhere, along with fans who found their spots in the stands. I dominated all my goals in the three assessment tests. I ran faster than ever, my vertical jump improved by over four inches, and my strength was my best yet. I was happy with my results because there were tons of scouts. I knew I had a chance, so after Pro Day I kept to my simplified lifestyle.

In May, on graduation day, my dad and stepmom

came out to Miami to watch me walk. I had finished the year with a 3.0 GPA and a Bachelor's Degree in Business Management. The day after I graduated, I officially signed with the San Francisco 49ers as a free agent. I headed back to my dorm, packed up everything I could, and got on a plane to California.

Boom! just like that everything changed. I was now a professional athlete. My journey had flowed beautifully into the next chapter of my life, which was the first time anything like that had happened. I hadn't forced anything, and because of that I was able to make a smooth transition to San Francisco.

Now, before I continue with this story, I wanted to throw in something about my past that I feel is quite important to add. After the abuse, when I moved in with my dad, the first thing he did was throw me into AAU basketball. He knew I needed an escape while dealing with my trauma, so basketball was a good way for me to cope. When I was with my abuser, we were at church four days a week, but when I moved in with my dad, every day after school was basketball practice. On weekends, there were tournaments. It was basketball nearly every day.

I joined AAU at a pretty early age, too. Most of the kids were two years older than me, and some were even playing for their sophomore basketball teams in high school. I was the runt of the bunch, and I knew it. On the court and in the weight room, I struggled to keep up. Besides learning skills I had never tried and dribbling coordination I had never seen, the worst of it all was the conditioning. Oh yes, the running was agonizing.

Coach Clarence's worst words he could ever say to us was always at the end of practice. "Get on the line." Conditioning was one of the worst things about basketball, but one of the most valuable things I took from sports. When we sprinted the court back and forth, we were all given a goal-time to beat. If one of us didn't beat our timer, we all ran again ... together. It kept us accountable. We couldn't control what anyone else did with their times, but we had to pay attention to doing our own part. Together we would all do this over and over until we all accomplished our goals as a team. What seemed like athletic torture was in fact a lesson. We had to hurt together in order to grow together.

And grow, we did. I couldn't be the player my teammates had to drag along. I wasn't about to hold my team back, so I pushed myself hard. I may have been younger and skinnier and weaker, but I wasn't going to be a stumbling block for my team's success. If I was going to benefit the team, then I needed to hone my skills daily. I learned drills faster, I memorized movement, I strengthened my stances, and I worked diligently on dribbling. I had to adapt as quickly and as efficiently as possible. I had to elevate myself in order to keep competing.

My middle school team won a tournament and I made the all-tournament team. With it, I received a shirt that had my name embroidered on it. I was so excited that I couldn't stop talking about it with my dad. I was so deeply happy.

When we got into the car, I said, "I can't wait to wear this to school this week and show everyone!"

As soon as both of our car doors were closed, my dad turned and looked at me, saying in a very calm voice, "Alright son, it's over now."

I stared back at him with a puzzled look, and didn't know how to respond.

"You got the award and you got to celebrate, but it's over now. How do you think your teammates will feel listening to you brag about your award at school?"

"Probably not good." I answered slowly, starting to understand what he was getting at.

"Probably not. Do you think this is the only all-tournament team you are going to make? Or will there be more?" He asked.

I said confidently, "I want to get more of them."

"Good. You got to enjoy it all the way to the car, but

now it's over. You should focus on the next one, not the last one. I am proud of you, Big Fella. You did great, but don't wear that shirt to school," Dad finished.

When I achieved one success, it was already over. Dad let me celebrate the moment, and he was proud of me, but it was just that, a moment. I hadn't finished the race. When you climb a ladder, you don't get to the top by staying in the middle. You keep climbing. And that's what he was teaching me. I wasn't done climbing.

So, after I graduated and after Pro Day, there was no time to celebrate my acceptance into the NFL. I had to keep climbing to the next rung, and then the next. I had to adapt and elevate myself in order to be ready for whatever was thrown at me. The next rung came at me fast.

Right away, I learned that if you wanted to be successful at the professional level, you had to be even more committed to the craft. There were no days off, lollygaggin', or shortcuts. I was going up against guys who had been playing at the top level for longer than I had played the sport, period. And I saw first-hand that the NFL wasn't just a sport, but it was also business.

In mere days I was learning things at practice that I never learned in college. I gained skills and techniques that were easy, aggressive, and adaptive. I caught on fast because I had to. I had to absorb everything if I wanted to stay with the team. I watched guys get cut for the smallest things, so I was deliberately aware of *everything* I did. I respected the sport, the league, and the craft.

I was absolutely fortunate that my first professional tight end coach was Eric Mangini. This guy already had so much success in the sport, and he knew it inside and out. He coached well, but he was also a great teacher. He taught me about how to understand the defensive side of things. This helped me adapt my skill as a tight end, and I learned hard and worked hard.

When our preseason game against the Houston Texans came around, I was ready. I scored a touchdown that game, and it felt amazing. I was able to contribute to my team as a rookie. Because I did so well in the preseason game, I was signed to the practice team. I was over the moon and I felt amazing.

Twenty minutes after signing, I was informed by Frank, my sports agent, that I had been cut from the 49ers. *What? Already?* I couldn't wrap my head around it. What had I done wrong? I couldn't figure it out. I didn't find out until later that someone else had signed to the team they hadn't expected to get, so they didn't need me. This was my first real experience with how the business-side of the NFL worked.

I was very emotional. All these years of hard work

had suddenly been taken away from me. I cried my eyes out as I packed up to head home. Everything had happened so fast, and in a blink of an eye ... it was all over. I just couldn't believe it. Ultimate high to ultimate low, just like that.

Right before I hit the road, I got another call from Frank. He told me, "Go back. They're going to re-sign you." Now I was really confused, but he didn't miss a beat. "And when you get back, don't hold a grudge. Move on." Though I didn't fully understand, I trusted what he told me. I mean, I was only 22 years old. What did I know at this level? Nothing!

He was right. Like nothing had ever happened, I was back attending practice. Our starting running back was Frank Gore, who also attended The University of Miami when they won a National Championship in 2001. He pulled me aside that first week and said something that really stuck with me, not just in sports, but in life. "Around here, you can't get complacent."

I knew every day I came to practice, I had to do my best. The other option was to get cut, and I already knew how that felt. I didn't want to experience it again. I had seen another guy get cut and not get a second chance. I did not want that to be me. If life was going to change in an instant, my mindset wasn't on the possibilities of my career ending, but about how each play and each step and each block was going to be my best. I began to transfer this mindset into how I lived the rest of my life as well outside of football.

Whenever I wasn't moving or blocking or catching, I was learning. And I learned from the best. The top dogs on the team were my role models, and they taught me more than I ever thought possible. Vernon Davis, Vance McDonald, Garret Celek, and Derek Carrier all took me under their wings. They were patient with me and treated me fairly, but they didn't baby me. I respected that. What they taught me in the sport I continue to demonstrate in life.

The majority of the time, I was on the practice squad and I was cool with that because I was still in the league. If I kept this up, maybe one day I'd get a shot at the big show. But I had to be patient, resilient, disciplined, and I had to keep giving my best. Then, all of a sudden, that opportunity came a knockin'.

During a regular season game, Vance and Vernon both got injured, and I was given my shot. We were playing the Seahawks. Our team ran a complicated game plan during run play, but like I had said, I learned hard and practiced hard. I had studied everything I could about our team and the opponents inside and out. I would fill in for the guys whenever they got hurt or needed breaks. I made sure the coaches and starters could depend on me. And depend on me they did.

I played six games as a rookie, and it felt amazing. When the season was over, I had four months off. It was crazy the amount of time I had available to myself. But I couldn't get complacent. I went back home to Sacramento and trained hard with the same trainer who helped me my sophomore year in college. I buckled down and focused. My mindset had changed, as did my philosophy. I had already made my dream of going to the NFL, now I was going to do whatever it took to stay there. Next season, I wanted to make more than the practice squad. I felt that if I could stay in the league, then I could be good enough for the next level.

By August, I was stronger and faster. My mind was set for active roster duties, but I had to prove my worth first at OTA's — Organized Team Activities. I didn't know who was watching, but I needed to stand out and show off my talent and progress. When we got through OTA's and into the preseason, we played the Texans again. This time I made 3 catches and took on my block responsibilities like a pro. I didn't play like a rookie anymore.

Shortly after, I was traded to the New England Patriots. It was humbling to know that the greatest coach of all time, Bill Belichick, was willing to give up something because he saw something great in me. I was now on the team that had just won the Super Bowl the previous season. This was it. The top level. The top program. And these athletes were the best of the best. A true meritocracy.

The coaches told me what they knew I was capable of and how I could best help the team. These coaches were the best, they knew everything football, so I did what they told me.

They had me starting with the practice squad. Coach Daboll told me to bring my creativity to the field. I was a versatile athlete, so that's what he wanted to see. And I absorbed everything. I learned about as many positions as I could on the offense. I studied the defenses. I gave myself homework. I wanted to live up to the Patriots' reputation. No way was I going to let these guys down.

Whenever I had the opportunity, I'd ask Tom Brady if he'd be willing to run routes with me. I knew that I had to initiate a connection with him. We were teammates, but I was still new, so I needed him to learn to trust me. I wanted him to see how I ran and how I turned into his passes. I wanted him to get used to throwing the ball to me, because if I ever had the chance to step onto the field, Brady needed to be comfortable and confident with me in there.

And guess what came a-knockin' again? That's right ... another opportunity. We were playing the Broncos on Sunday Night Football. After a teammate got injured, I was put onto the field. I made my first professional football career catch, and it was thrown by Tom Brady. Hundreds of passes, thousands of hours of committing to the craft, all for this one moment.

The next game, I started as full back against the Texans. I had done it, I had not only made it to the active roster from the practice squad, but I now had my first professional start in the NFL. My first play was to cut-block JJ Watts. I'll never forget it. Everything was falling into place. I was where I was meant to be.

Two weeks later, it was Christmas. A few teammates and I attended a Christmas dinner at the home of another teammate. It felt like family, all of us together. Our spirits were high. Then, as we sat down to eat dinner, I got a phone call. I had been cut from the team. I was no longer a New England Patriot.

The coaches told me they were needing a corner and finally got one, but they reassured me they were going to re-sign me to the practice squad. Well, knowing how the NFL worked, nothing was concrete or set in stone. And before I could sign back up with the Patriots, I had been claimed off waivers by the Chargers. I flew out to San Diego for the final game of the season.

The Patriots went on to win the Super Bowl the following year. I spent the last two seasons of my career with the Chargers, but I didn't see this as a consequence or a demotion. This was just more life had to offer with more opportunities. And the Chargers were going to get my best.

It also gave me the opportunity to learn from my favorite NFL football player, Antonio Gates. This guy was the athlete I always wanted to be like. He was already fourteen years into the NFL, and he was possibly the greatest tight end in all NFL history. I didn't only respect him as an athlete, but also as a human being.

He had been a college basketball player just like I had wanted to be, and then went undrafted as a free agent into the NFL. I learned so much from him, and I was amazed by his on-field and off-field knowledge, intelligence, and wisdom. He taught me simplicity over complication when it came to strategy and technique — work smarter not harder. It humbled me to watch him and know I was good enough to be on this level. I was grateful to be around him, and I was even there when he tied the most touchdowns in history for a tight end.

Going into my fourth season, I had spent six solid weeks in Miami, training my butt off. While there, I found out that I was somehow still missing one college credit. I couldn't understand how that was possible, and why it was just coming to my attention *now*, but the school told me that during my junior year, I hadn't earned enough credits to get my degree, so I was one class short. I remembered that was the year I was at a 1.8 GPA, when life was at a low point, and I had dropped any class I struggled with. Apparently I had dropped one too many, and now I needed to complete this one, single credit in order to earn my degree. Despite the fact that it hadn't been noticed right away, the fault was mine and mine alone, and I had to fix it. Rather than complain or make excuses, I did what I needed to do. I took a negotiation class and earned an A, allowing me to officially graduate again.

The minute I was done fixing my school problem, I was back to work. I trained hard and studied hard. This was going to be a big year for me. I felt I could make the active roster this year, even though I hadn't contributed much last season. But this season was going to be different. I put in the work and I was ready to move forward with the Chargers.

Four days into camp, we were having a joint practice with the Los Angeles Rams. I was running a post route, planted my foot wrong, and went down. I had torn my meniscus in my knee. I knew I was hurt, and would once again need to take time to heal, but I had no idea that this seemingly small injury was going to be the end of my career in the NFL.

# 43

# BE DISCIPLINED RATHER THAN MOTIVATED

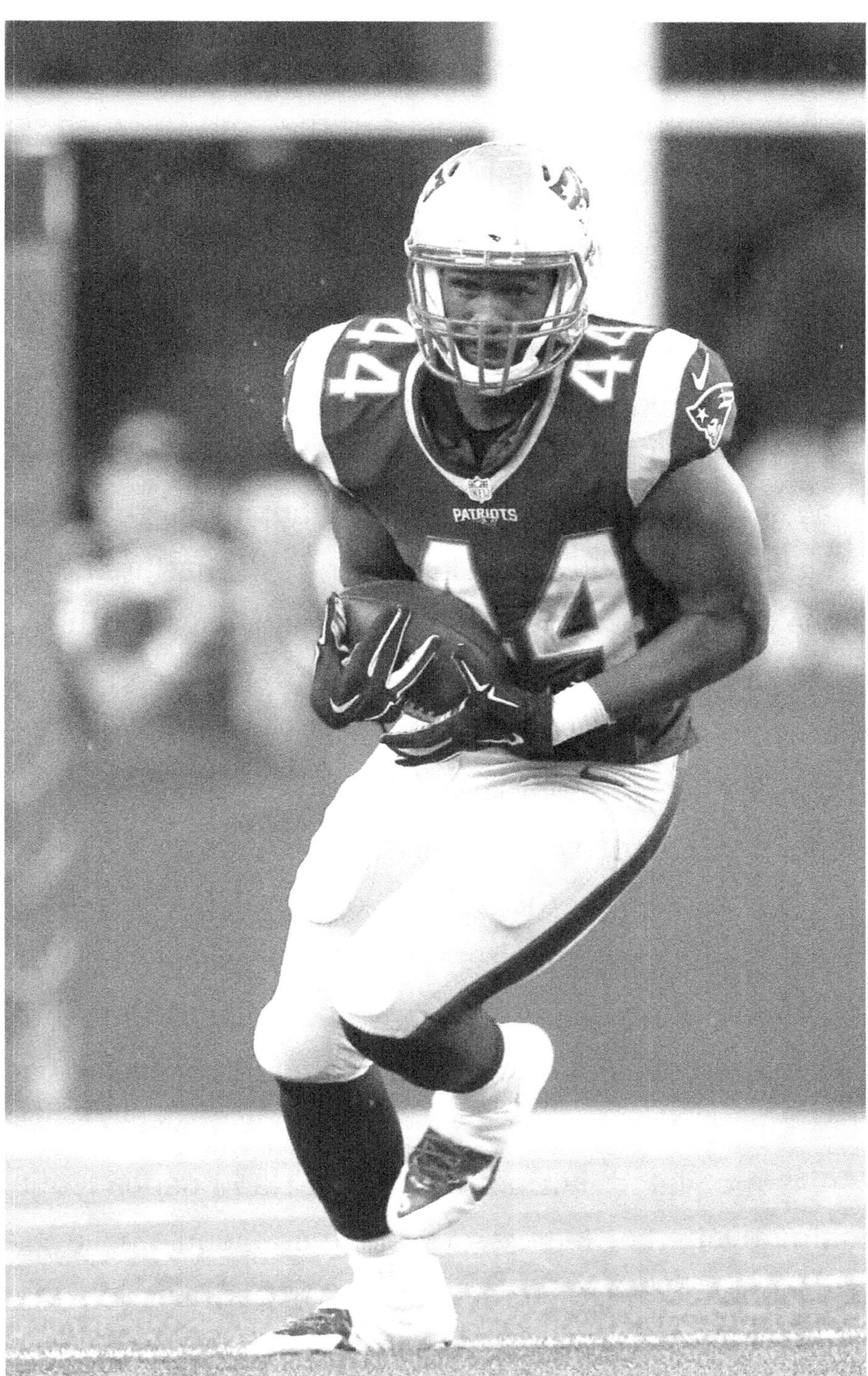

had a decision to make now, and these choices would have serious ramifications in the end. The meniscus is a wedge-shaped cartilage that acts as a cushion between the thigh bone and shin bone. The doctors gave me two options. I could take out the torn meniscus and only have to recover for six weeks or I could have surgery to repair it, be placed on Injured Reserve, and recovery would be six months. The first option sounded great because I'd get to play again before the season ended, but it was guaranteed that my body would develop arthritis in that area of the knee ten years down the road. Also, knowing how the NFL functioned, I would have almost certainly been cut the minute I returned. Not many coaches would want to take a risk to have an athlete playing with a removed meniscus; there'd be too many potential issues to deal with.

I went with the second option. For the next six months after the surgery, I disciplined myself more than ever. I continued to work on my upper body. I hated that the surgery was slowing me down and holding me back, but I made the decision to just focus on moving forward. I was motivated, but not every day. Had I depended just on motivation or feeling inspired, then I would have been disappointed. I had learned from my past mistakes that I had to stay goal-oriented despite my emotional state.

I've learned that motivation requires reasons to do something. It usually requires feelings of inspiration and a certain degree of excitement to get something done. I can tell you that when I woke up in the mornings and looked at my knee, I didn't feel inspired. I knew in the back of my mind that the NFL may not let me back in because of this injury. I had many reasons why I needed to keep moving forward, but I also had many reasons why I just wanted to stop. Motivation on its own is not enough. Let me explain.

Take New Year's resolutions for example. Many of us have this silly habit of waiting for the new year to roll around to motivate us to make a lifestyle change — quit smoking, start a diet, exercise more, find happiness, get better with money, go back to school, and the list can go on. These are all good intentions to make good changes in life, and we have good reasons to strive for these new goals. It's awesome and amazing and we're motivated by wanting these changes. So, then, why do over 70% of New Year Resolutions fail by February? Why do we restart these resolutions year after year after year? We have the motivation, the excitement, we have the reasons, and the willingness.

But we lack discipline. With New Year resolutions, we may have reasons behind our goals, but we also find reasons (excuses) to stop them. And trust me, excuses are very easy to find. I have a question: if we have lifestyle changes we want to make so badly, then why do we wait until the New Year to get started? Why not start now? There's no better time than now to make good changes and start new, positive habits, right?

Well, there's more to it than that. Let's look at the difference between motivation and discipline. Sure, we've gone through this before, but it's important to address it again. Being motivated to accomplish a goal requires numerous things to work towards something like: the willingness to do it, a desire to do it, a reason to do it, and having an interest to do it. So what happens when we are willing to wake up at 4:00 a.m. to stick to our morning walks or writing sessions? What if we desire sleeping in instead of getting up? What if we find reasons or excuses to stop working on these new habits? Maybe we tell ourselves we'll get back into it tomorrow? What if we just aren't interested in our goal anymore? These are easy thoughts (or seeds) that get planted in our brain, and they don't require much attention to grow. They're like a weed in our garden, and we choose to pull them out or keep them there.

Okay, so now let's look at what's required to be disciplined. It's simply defined as demonstrating self-control in how we behave, work, and function. There are no reasons or feelings or desires to be disciplined. Being disciplined is a choice — to have control or not. To do or to do not. To be or not to be.

If we want what is best for us or healthiest for us, it requires intense discipline to break those bad habits and to pull out overgrown weeds of negative thinking. Discipline doesn't require other people's opinions, either. If *you* want to make a change in *your* life, then *you* are the one that has to change, inside and out. It's about self-control. So, while motivation can be helpful, discipline is the only thing that's going to get you out of bed *despite* the excuses. Discipline says "this is the only thing that will get me to my goal, no matter how I feel today."

I could have chosen to remove my meniscus and get back in the NFL after six weeks, but like I said, the guaranteed outcomes and consequences would have been a lifelong battle of arthritis and further surgeries and injections. I had to discipline myself and have the surgery, taking the slower, but hopefully more effective route towards my goal. Every day, my focus was to return to the NFL as the league's best blocking tight end. I hit the gym three days a week while recovering and healing, focusing on my upper body strength. In those six months, my bench press went from 290 pounds to 390 pounds. I didn't want to take time off because complacency will make your goals unreachable. Do you think I was motivated towards that goal? Sure, but not every day. Some days I just needed a break, so instead of being complacent on my days off I filled it with more creative outlets.

I started taking both voice acting and regular acting classes. Throughout my life, I'd been told that I have a voice for radio, so I challenged those statements and put my money where my mouth was ... literally. I have a naturally deep voice, so I took time to tap into it more, to build up new skills. This was something that interested me and led me to an opportunity to do some sportscasting for a while. I was willing to work on new talents and see what they had to offer, so I stuck with it for a while. Even acting class was an enjoyable experience, learning how to express my words through facial expressions and body language. It was a new form of communication I wanted to improve. This was also very inspiring to me, but neither were long term goals. They were just interesting ways to broaden my scope of experience, so I eventually stepped away from them. It was awesome trying new things, and I have no regrets putting my time into these practices. My story isn't over yet, so who knows? Maybe I'll put these learning experiences to even more good use someday!

We all need to care about what we want in life and how we can better help people by making ourselves better first. I was disciplined during my recovery because I wanted to be strong, and I was going to use that strength to be a better blocker when I got put back on with a team. I took voice acting lessons so I could use my voice to communicate and inspire others. If you have a goal, be deliberate about achieving that goal, and if/when you make mistakes in the process, don't just brush them to the side. Acknowledge them and deliberately change yourself in such a way that you don't make the same mistakes again. It's like the statue David. Michelangelo was given a single block of white marble before starting his masterpiece. The vision of David was already inside, but the artist had to carve, mold, shape, and chip away at that block until all that was left was David. Michelangelo worked diligently on his vision. He already saw David inside the block, and after two years of committed discipline, he accomplished this breathtaking work of art.

We are the block of marble *and* we are the artist. We all have visions for ourselves and where we want to be in the future. We all have, at some time or another, envisioned ourselves as attractive, confident, strong, wealthy, famous, happy, successful, smart, athletic, accepted, appreciated, desired, fulfilled, and loved. We all have goals, hopes, and aspirations. But it is all in the hands of our creative "Michelangelo" side, the one that chips away and carves the vision out of the block. It's messy, it's exhausting, and it's time consuming, but in the end it will be magnificent. You will be magnificent. You already are. If you can find the courage to search for the possibilities within yourself, then start chipping away.

## OVERTIME REFLECTION

- In what areas of your life are you very disciplined? Where do you lack discipline?

- How can you purposely build momentum in small ways?

- What bad habits can you change to be more disciplined?

# 44

## WISDOM COMES FROM EXPERIENCE

As I was getting close to the end of my recovery, I was already doing sportscasting on the radio for NBC, keeping my feet wet in the sport as my healing improved. Then, finally, I was able to go free agent and get back on the list. I was ready to show off my new strength, and I was ready to rock 'n' roll. The New England Patriots heard I was back and took an interest. I flew out and met with their doctors. They took a few MRIs of my knee to see if it was safe for me to play on. I felt good. I felt confident and hopeful. Things were going great, so when I went back to the hotel and my agent called with bad news, I wasn't ready for it. "Asante, based off the MRIs, the doctors said the repair didn't take, and because of that the Patriots aren't going to sign you."

That was a heavy blow to my spirit and an opportunity for my historical lies to resurface. I began to feel valueless. After the call, I kind of went dormant inside my head. There was a numbness inside of me, a void of emptiness. As I moved through the airport to get on my flight home, I once again felt like a ghost in a crowd. I wasn't processing any thoughts and time just moved along as if I didn't exist.

On the plane, as I was stowing my carry-on in the overhead compartment, a woman recognized the significance of the security straps still attached to my bag. They gave professional athletes clearance into the stadiums.

She spoke up, "Hey, I know you. Don't you play for the Patriots?"

This was not the time for me to have this conversation with a stranger. "No, ma'am. I don't."

"Yes, you do. Yes, you do."

My stomach was churning and I was boiling by this point. I didn't want to admit to a stranger that I hadn't made the team, but as I turned to say just that, I recognized the woman. She was Coach Belichick's girlfriend. I figured she had a right to know, so instead of letting my feelings get the best of me, I simply told her, "I didn't pass my physical assessment. They wouldn't have me." And then filled in the unhappy details.

After the flight, I caught up with her again and asked her to pass on a message to Coach Belichick. "Would you please tell him that I appreciated him thinking about me? Please, tell them thank you for bringing me back and giving me the opportunity to be a Patriot." She agreed she would and we went our separate ways. As much as everything hurt, I was still genuinely grateful to this man for the opportunities he had made possible.

When I got home, I sought out doctors to get a second opinion about my knee. Only one doctor gave me hope. He said I hadn't worked on its durability yet. I hadn't seen if it could handle anything strenuous. So, I spent time at home running routes, making cuts left and right, sprinting and turning. While experimenting on my knee, other teams had reached out and encouraged me to contact them if things worked out.

But sadly, when I did finally make it to the point where I could reach out to those same teams, there was no response. Three months of radio silence. It was all over. And I knew it.

Now what?

Those two simple words, that one question, tormented me for months. It was tough not knowing what was going to happen, *if* something was going to happen. Midway through football season, I knew my time in the NFL was cut short. I didn't want to waste time chasing something that didn't want to be pursued, but now I had come to a fork in the road. One path had ended, and another one was about to begin. And the thing that bothered me most, was the terror I was feeling about this new, unknown path.

I thought long and hard about what I needed to do next. Should I keep trying to get back into the NFL? Do I take a chance at radio and sportscasting? Do I pursue voice acting or an acting career? I spent a lot of time searching for the answers to these questions, but one thing was very clear. Football was not my purpose. I had worked as hard as I could, and I had played football well, but that was over now, and I was still here. So, what was my new purpose? How did I see myself in the world if I didn't have football anymore?

I started testing the waters, getting new jobs and trying out new things. For a while, I ran a photo booth company for parties. At one event, there was a huge line of people waiting to use our photo booth, but as I stood there, wearing that fake smile, deep down I didn't feel happy. I didn't really enjoy this, so I moved on.

I then got hired on at a wholesale investment company that bought and flipped houses. My job was to cold call investors and offer a fee to purchase and flip their businesses, where I learned something else about myself. The confidence and bravado it took to have these phone calls over and over and over again with investors that wanted nothing to do with me did not exist. I watched my coworkers call investors nine different times with the same charismatic voice, each time getting hung up on. One of my coworker's numbers got blocked so much he ended up using other people's phones to keep nagging the investor. And yet somehow, he maintained that same course of positive attitude each phone call. It was astonishing. He had something I wanted to learn, so I got to know him better.

We were having a conversation about life one day, and he told me he was from the Chicago suburban area. As a kid he had been playing soccer in his basement and had accidentally busted out a basement light. My initial response was, "Man, I bet your dad beat you for that."

He just looked at me for a moment, and then replied, "No, but he was pissed." And that's when I realized something about myself.

My abuser would have beaten me severely for such an offense. I suddenly made the connection between this man's confidence and bravado, and my lack of those skills. As a kid, and through the years of abuse, I always second guessed myself because of the consequences that were to follow. This guy had busted the light in his dad's basement and he was able to laugh about the story. I couldn't do that. Throughout my whole life after my abuse, I wasn't able to make confident choices without hesitating. I didn't handle rejection well, and I also had an empty spot inside my heart where something was missing.

I knew this wasn't the job for me, but I didn't give up on it. I was learning more about myself, and strengthening myself in new ways. I had created good habits not to be complacent, so I continued waking up early and showing up to work early. I made my phone calls and never missed a day of work. I was a loyal employee, but over time I just wasn't able to keep up to my employer's expectations, and they let me go. I didn't miss the job, but I was thankful for the experience it provided me.

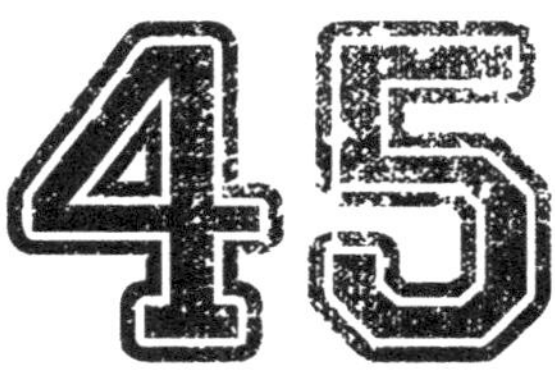

# DREAMS AFTER DISAPPOINTMENT

There was a point after my injury when I reached out to my abuser. I invited her out to dinner because I wanted to bury the hatchet. She showed up late, and unfortunately our conversation didn't really surprise me. When I brought up the abuse, she still felt justified in how she treated me. There was no apology or regret from her. But somehow, even though we didn't resolve anything, I was glad I had done it. I was ready to move on with my life, even if she wasn't ready to acknowledge she had done anything wrong. I had done what I could do.

After this, I took the time to really process my past, present, and future. I started seeing a therapist who really helped me progress. I knew I needed to meet with somebody professional. I had started having suicidal thoughts that were directly linked with my unresolved trauma as a child. I knew I had to seek out help beyond myself. I had trouble feeling whole even though I was outwardly a pretty confident guy. My entire life of second guessing myself kept bringing me back to my childhood, and I became aware that my mindset as a kid carried over into my adulthood. I had never addressed those mental barriers, and because of it I was still experiencing the same challenges I had as a kid. So, when I got let go from the investment company, I saw it as a gift. Being cut from the NFL was still fresh, so getting let go from a job was also hard on a guy rebuilding his confidence. But now that I was unemployed, I had room in my life to work on the things from my past that needed addressing.

With the help of my therapist, I began working on myself the next couple months, writing and journaling my life out like a story. I addressed thoughts, feelings, struggles, and barriers I hadn't overcome yet even as an adult. I was relearning who I was and who I wanted to be, basically starting the whole process all over again. I needed to rediscover myself, and at times it was quite painful.

Then, two months later, the COVID-19 pandemic hit, and more insecurities resurfaced again. Being at home I started thinking more about my past and what I had gone through as a child. There were so many painful thoughts I had buried for so very long, and when quarantine occurred, I was basically forced into addressing those pains head on. That's when I realized something.

I had to accept things as they were, because despite the darkness, my experiences had led me to the person I was today. Without the trials, I would never have learned all those crucial lessons from my dad, which later became important tools to help me grow into an athlete. I had to let go of expectations of how I thought things *should* go or how I thought people *should* act.

This book was never meant to be an "I'm right and you're wrong" story for my abuser. It also isn't about the glamour of being an NFL athlete. In fact, it's just the opposite. In chapter 1, I said we all have a story. Well, this is simply *my* story. I chose to write it because I wanted people to know that we all go through stuff. I feel that if there is even one person out there who can improve the outcome of their life from reading this, then writing this book was worth it. It's not easy for me to be open and vulnerable about my past, but that's the exact reason why I felt I needed to write it.

People often want to keep the messy parts of their life to themselves to hide it and bury it and move on. Well, it's not easy to do that because it follows you. I'm on my way out of my twenties and I'm still hashing things out with my past. But one thing I am learning is that facing and accepting, and even sometimes talking about the mess, helps me find the bright spots in it that are leading me to the future I'm meant for.

I just had a conversation with someone while in the middle of writing this book, and we talked about my struggle to gain a sense of confidence. The guy commented, "It's not self-confidence you're looking for. You already got that. It's self-worth you're seeking. Think of it like a football player. Self-confidence represents the shoulder pads, jersey, helmet, and extra accessories players wear. They look cool, walk cool, and fans want to be just like them. But self-worth represents the athlete under the pads. It's the athlete that brings value to each play and to the team, not the appearance. Asante, you've always had the confidence, you just need to see your worth. Once you see it, you'll realize the value you can offer the world with your story."

We all have a past and we all have a future. We all make choices, good and bad. Kent, the Olympic diver, said, "It's about knowing and accepting that you will fail in life; guaranteed. The point is not failing, but how you recover. You can take so much from failure and learn from it, or simply stop moving forward."

We all have a path, whether you believe it or not. And we all have confidence in some area in our life. The right question is do we have self-worth? Ask yourself that question. Do you feel you have value to offer? Do you have value to invest in yourself? It's not about what you can obtain from the world, but what you can offer it.

People are who they are, which is fine. They will make their own choices. People's philosophies will be different than yours; they will choose to perceive the world and how they fit inside of it in their own way. You can't change them, only yourself. We can want what's best for other people, but sometimes people don't want what's best for the world. And that's pretty hard to accept. Just affect what you are able.

I had to learn to accept things for how they were ... like my past. I had to let go of the expectation that my abuser would be accountable for what she had done to me. Once I was able to do that, it was like I had a bigger revelation.

I realized there are a lot of other people dealing with similar struggles. I finally became aware that there were kids and adults out there who could relate and understand the pain my eleven-year-old self had gone through. And they needed to know that they aren't the only ones. And what they were/are dealing with is something they *will* get through. They needed to know that they could steer out of the storm like I had done.

Whoever you are, with whatever you are going through, be encouraged. It won't stay this way forever if you don't let it. It won't always be an obstacle. Everything you want to achieve is still possible, as long as you're still willing to keep moving forward. Don't hold on tightly to the past, just keep your eyes on the future and push forward. A dream without a journey is just a dream. There is a dream embedded inside of you, just waiting for you to pursue it. Take the first step.

# OVERTIME REFLECTION

- As we near the end of this book, what has shifted inside of you?

- Where do you hope this journey will take you, and what are you most excited about?

- Are you ready to be great?

# APPENDIX I

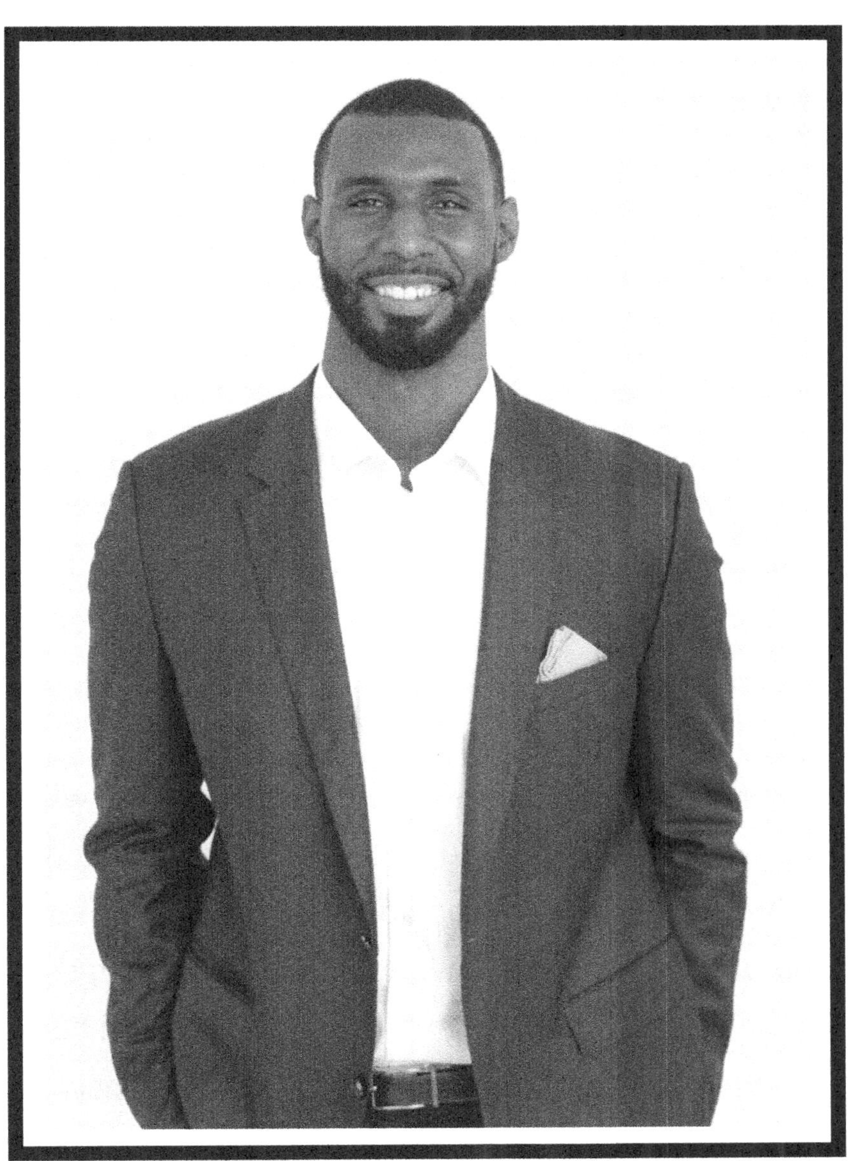

# Asante's Letter to the Readers
## (Why Am I Doing This?)

*Dear dreamer,*

I want you to know that you are capable of anything you set your mind to, regardless of what you have been through. Any and all obstacles you have had to deal with in your life are a part of what makes your story incredible. You, and only you, are able to handle what lies ahead on your journey. Each challenge you face only makes you stronger and better prepared to handle anything that life throws at you. It won't be easy, I assure you, but you are unbreakable.

**Believe in yourself.**

Whatever you decide to pursue, do it with an unshakable self belief. You will face rejections along the way, but don't let that stop you. No one else will believe in you until you do. You have to be your own biggest fan. You gain confidence through putting in hours and hours of work. It takes 10,000 hours of practice to be considered a master at anything. Put in the time and your confidence will grow.

## Keep your head up.

You will make mistakes along the way, we all do. No mistake that you, or anyone else, makes is the end of the world. This is an opportunity for you to learn and grow. Pick yourself up and do your best to not make the same mistakes twice. If you know better then you can do better.

## Make friends.

The journey is long, so make sure you have good people around you. Surround yourself with people who encourage you to be yourself, and help you grow. Be a great friend to them as well, no one succeeds alone.

## Dream big.

Whatever you enjoy doing, try to do it at the highest level possible. I want you to know that it is possible, as long as you are putting in the time and you are fully committed. It doesn't matter what other people think about your dreams, they are yours and yours alone. Reach for something that gets you excited, and even a little scared. Keep putting one foot in front of the other and you will get to your destination in perfect timing.

## Do your best.

Give your best effort to everything you do. Many things in life are out of your control, but you are always in control of the effort you give. You know when you are doing your best, and you know when you aren't. As long as you are always doing your best, your best always gets better.

You can do anything in life as long as you believe you can. Stay focused on what you want, and keep working through the dark. You got this.

*From Your Fan,*

**Asante Cleveland**